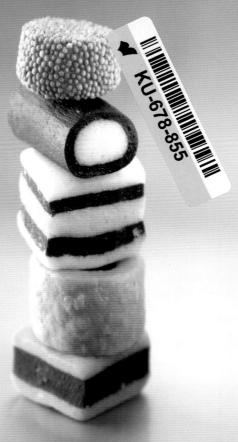

KU-678-855

# contents

## ACKNOWLEDGEMENTS

The *BESTMEDICINE Simple Guides* team is very grateful to a number of people who have made this project possible. In particular we'd like to thank Anne Taylor, Jane Cassidy, Caroline Delasalle and Amelie (5 months). Thank you to Ben for his endless enthusiasm, energy and creativity, to Molly (7) and George (5) and of course to Hetta. Julie and Rob who went far beyond the call of duty and Julie's ability to put pages together for hours on end was hugely inspiring. Thank you also to Gemma Groves of Bodyclock for the loan of a TENS machine *www.bodyclock.co.uk*

### A Simple Guide to your Health Service

Emma Catherall          Co-ordinator

### Advisory Panel

Richard Stevens         GP
Carole Bradshaw         Physiotherapist
Michael Gum             Pharmacist
John Chater             Binley's health and care
                        information specialist
                        *www.binleys.com*

The
Patients
Association

# a simple guide to
# **back pain**

**BESTMEDICINE** Health Handbooks

A Simple Guide to Back Pain
First published – September 2005

**Published by**
**CSF Medical Communications Ltd**
1 Bankside, Lodge Road, Long Hanborough
Oxfordshire, OX29 8LJ, UK
T +44 (0)1993 885370 F +44 (0)1993 881868
*enquiries@bestmedicine.com*
*www.bestmedicine.com*
*www.csfmedical.com*

**Editor** Dr Eleanor Bull
**Medical Editor** Dr Graham Archard
**Creative Director & Project Manager** Julia Potterton
**Designer** Lee Smith
**Layout** Julie Smith
**Publisher** Stephen I'Anson

© CSF Medical Communications Ltd 2005

ISBN: 1-905466-01-3

*BESTMEDICINE* is a trademark of CSF Medical Communications Ltd

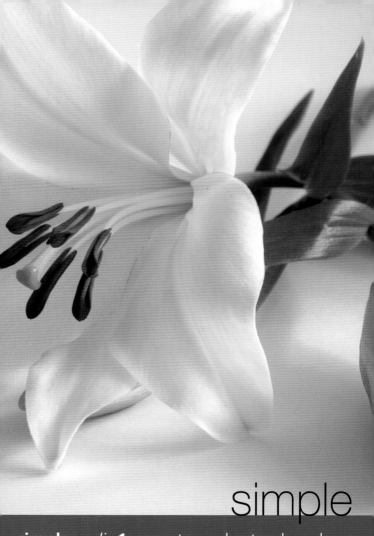

simple

**simple** *adj.* **1.** easy to understand or do: *a simple problem.* **2.** plain; unadorned: *a simple dress.* **3.** Not combined or complex: *a simple mechanism.* **4.** Unaffected or unpretentious: *although he became famous he remained a simple man.* **5.** sincere; frank: *a simple explanation was readily accepted.* **6.** (*prenominal*) without additions or modifications: *the witness told the simple truth.*

## ABOUT THE AUTHOR

### ELEANOR BULL

*Eleanor graduated from King's College London with a BSc Honours degree in Pharmacology and then completed a PhD in Neuroscience at the University of Nottingham. As well as publishing her own research work internationally, Eleanor has written for numerous publications in the* BESTMEDICINE *series. She now lives in the West of Ireland.*

## ABOUT THE EDITOR

### GRAHAM ARCHARD

*Graham Archard is a GP who lives and practises in Dorset. He is the Vice Chairman of the Royal College of General Practitioners and is chair of the College's clinical services network. He is also joint Professional Executive Committee Chair and clinical governance lead of the South and East Dorset Primary Care Trust.*

**TRISHA MACNAIR**

*Doctor and BBC Health Journalist*

Getting involved in managing your own medical condition – or helping those you love or care for to manage theirs – is a vital step towards keeping as healthy as possible. Whilst doctors, nurses and the rest of your healthcare team can help you with expert advice and guidance, nobody knows your body, your symptoms and what is right for *you* as well as you do.

There is no long-term (chronic) medical condition or illness that I can think of where the person concerned has absolutely no influence at all on their situation. The way you choose to live your life, from the food you eat to the exercise you take, will impact upon your disease, your well-being and how able you are to cope. You are in charge!

Being involved in making choices about your treatment helps you to feel in control of your problems, and makes sure you get the help that you really need. Research clearly shows that when people living with a chronic illness take an active role in looking after themselves, they can bring about significant improvements in their illness and vastly improve the quality of life they enjoy. Of course, there may be occasions when you feel particularly unwell and it all seems out of your control. Yet most of the time there are plenty of things that you can do in order to reduce the negative effects that your condition can have on your life. This way you feel as good as possible and may even be able to alter the course of your condition.

So how do you gain the confidence and skills to take an active part in managing your condition, communicate with health professionals and work through sometimes worrying and emotive issues? The answer is to become better informed. Reading about your problem, talking to others who have been through similar experiences and hearing what the experts have to say will all help to build-up your understanding and help you to take an active role in your own health care.

*BESTMEDICINE Simple Guides* provide an invaluable source of help, giving you the facts that you need in order to understand the key issues and discuss them with your doctors and other professionals involved in your care. The information is presented in an accessible way but without neglecting the important details. Produced independently and under the guidance of medical experts *A Simple Guide to Back Pain* is an evidence-based, balanced and up-to-date review that I hope you will find enables you to play an active part in the successful management of your condition.

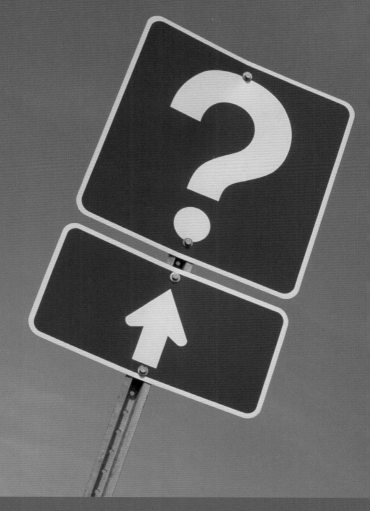

# what happens normally?

# WHY IS IT IMPORTANT THAT WE FEEL PAIN?

Pain is our body's way of telling us that something is wrong. It works as an alarm system, a signal to tell us to stop doing something that may be harmful to us, and in this way protects us from dangerous situations. For this reason, pain should always be taken seriously.

Pain is a subjective feeling – it is influenced by personal opinion.

Our ability to withstand pain depends a lot on the mood we are in, our personality and the circumstances under which our pain occurs. In the heat of the moment (e.g. during an exciting football match), we may be able to override our feelings of pain to get the job done.

In the FA Cup final of 1956, the Manchester City goalkeeper, Bert Trautmann, broke his neck 15 minutes before the end of the match, yet he continued to play and saw his team clinch victory.

**OUR NERVOUS SYSTEM**

Nerve cells can transmit nervous impulses at 225 miles per hour.

Pain gets on our nerves, quite literally. Our perception of pain is controlled by our nervous system, the part of our bodies that records and distributes information throughout the body. Our nervous system is in two parts, the central nervous system and the peripheral nervous system.

The smallest unit of the nervous system is the nerve cell or neuron. These are highly specialised structures that are able to conduct

*We cannot learn without pain.*
Aristotle

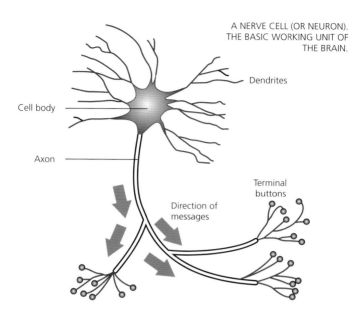

A NERVE CELL (OR NEURON).
THE BASIC WORKING UNIT OF
THE BRAIN.

Dendrites

Cell body

Axon

Terminal
buttons

Direction of
messages

messages to and from the brain as fast-moving nerve impulses (electrical signals). Nerve cells communicate with each other via their dendrites, spindly extensions that act as antennae and gather information for the nerve cell to deal with. Nerves themselves are made up of bundles of the axons of the nerve cells. They transmit electrical nerve impulses between the peripheral and central nervous systems. To look at it another way, nerves are the electrical wiring of the body and the brain and spinal cord are the nerve centre – the mission control of pain perception.

The central nervous system is made up of the brain and the spinal cord.

The peripheral nervous system comprises the nerves that transmit sensations between the central nervous system and the rest of the body.

*Pain is inevitable. Suffering is optional.*
Dalai Lama

3

## WHAT DO OUR BACKS DO FOR US?

Our backs are an essential part of who we are. Without them, we would be unable to stand, walk, twist, turn, bend or lift. We use our backs in almost every activity of daily living. Therefore, when we experience pain in our backs, we must take it seriously.

The term 'back' describes the trunk of the body from below the neck, right down to the tailbone. The upper back is called the thoracic spine and the lower back is the lumbar spine. The back is made up of bone, muscle and other types of tissue. Thirty-three small bones called vertebrae (shaped like irregular rings) are stacked on top of each other to form the spine which supports the weight of the body and houses and protects the spinal cord. Topped by the skull, the spinal column sits in a large bony bowl called the pelvis. The tailbone or coccyx (*pronounced kok-six*), is a set of fused vertebrae at the base of the spine and serves no real function.

The vertebrae, which give our back flexibility, are stacked on top of each other and connected by discs at the front and by facet joints at the back. The discs that separate the vertebrae provide cushioning and act as shock absorbers. Facet joints (found only in the lower back) are cup-shaped surfaces that form movable joints with our hips. At each of the vertebrae, nerves branch out to the rest of the body. Tough ligaments help to bind the vertebrae together and strengthen the back.

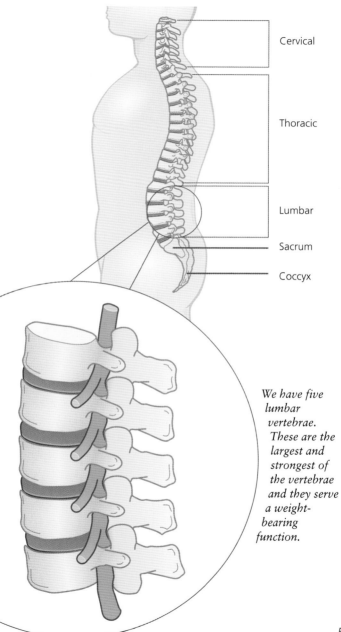

Cervical

Thoracic

Lumbar

Sacrum

Coccyx

*We have five lumbar vertebrae. These are the largest and strongest of the vertebrae and they serve a weight-bearing function.*

5

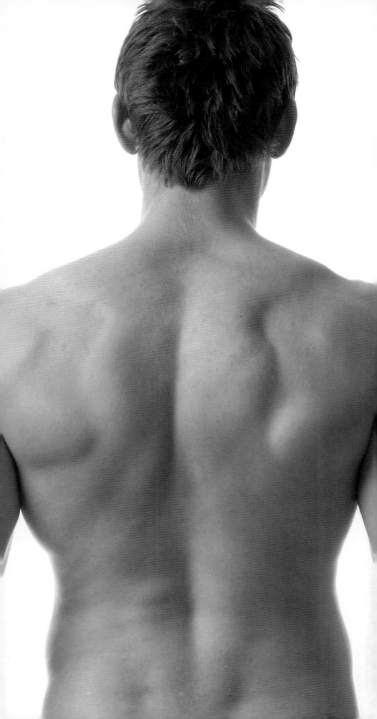

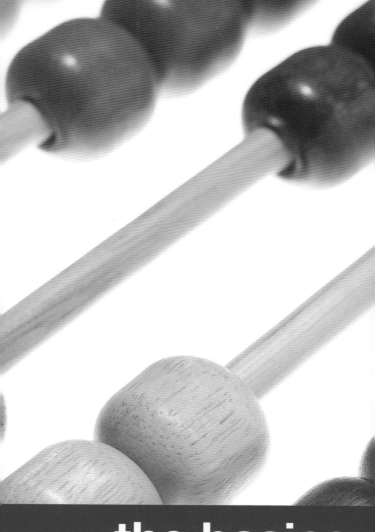

# the basics

# BACK PAIN – THE BASICS

Back pain is not a disease in itself. It is a collection of symptoms that signifies something is wrong. If managed properly, back pain can resolve within a matter of days or weeks.

### WHAT IS PAIN?

We all know what pain means to us but it is often a very difficult thing to describe. Pain can be defined as an unpleasant sensation that occurs when we experience trauma or damage to our bodies. Pain may be aching, burning, throbbing, shooting, tingling or stabbing.

### WHEN DOES PAIN BECOME A PROBLEM?

Pain becomes a problem to us when it affects the way in which we live our lives. This is usually because it lasts a long time, or becomes **chronic**.

### DIFFERENT TYPES OF PAIN

There are three major types of pain – acute nociceptive, inflammatory and neuropathic.
- Bee stings and twisted ankles are examples of nociceptive pain. This is pain that occurs following damage to the bones, joints, skin or soft tissue of the body.
- Pain in the joints caused by rheumatoid arthritis is an example of inflammatory pain.

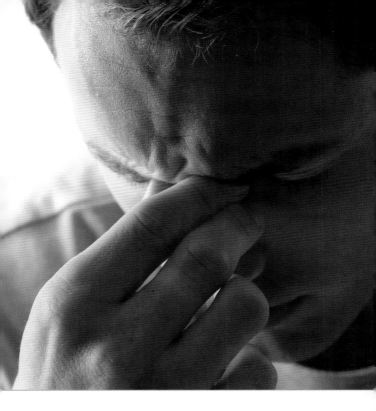

■ Headaches and trapped nerves can be neuropathic in their origin. Neuropathic pain usually follows damage to nerve tissues.

Pain is also described in terms of how long it lasts. **Acute**, or short-lasting, pain is pain that lasts for less than 8 weeks and **chronic**, or long-lasting, pain generally lasts for more than 2 months. This is true no matter where the pain is, or what's causing the pain.

Acute pain is important because it warns us of the potential for or extent of an injury, allowing us to adapt our behaviour accordingly. In contrast, chronic pain doesn't serve a protective, or adaptive, purpose. Instead, it disrupts our sleep and our normal way of living.

9

### WHAT IS BACK PAIN?

Most back pain is **simple back pain** (or backache), pain that is linked to the way in which the bones, ligaments and muscles of the back work together. This is usually pain that:

- occurs as a result of lifting, bending or straining
- comes and goes
- most often affects the lower back
- does not usually signify any permanent damage.

Some back pain is linked to **nerve root pain**. This is much less common than simple back pain and accounts for about 5% of back pain cases. Nerve root pain is usually caused by compression of the start of a nerve as it leaves the spinal cord. Herniated discs (commonly, but incorrectly, called 'slipped discs') are one cause of nerve root pain.

Sciatica (*pronounced Si-attica*) – in which the sciatic nerve that runs down the legs becomes irritated – is a relatively common example of nerve root pain.

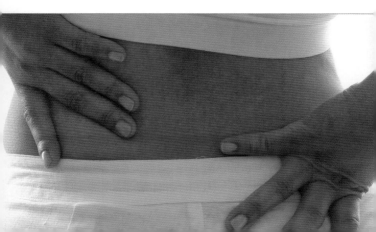

## SYMPTOMS OF BACK PAIN

Pain itself is a very subjective feeling and its perceived severity is highly influenced by personal opinion and the circumstances under which it occurs. The symptoms of back pain can vary hugely from one person to the next. They include:

- aching
- stiffness
- numbness
- weakness
- tingling (pins and needles).

Coughing or sneezing can often make back pain much worse by causing the muscles of the back to go into painful spasm. The pain may start in your back but may travel elsewhere. It often goes into the buttocks, but may go further down the leg and even into the foot.

If pain gets really bad, or lasts for a long time, you may experience:

- difficulty passing urine
- difficulty sleeping
- sexual problems
- depression.

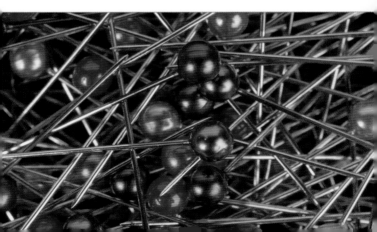

## WHAT CAUSES BACK PAIN?

There are a whole host of reasons why you
might experience back pain. Your pain might
be a consequence of everyday life (such as bad
posture whilst driving or when sitting at your
desk) or, less often, it might be as a result of
some underlying disease. The majority of cases
of back pain are linked to simple mechanical
problems, less than 5% signify nerve root pain
and less than 2% reflect serious spinal
pathology.

Pathology is the study
of diseases, their
causes and their
consequences.

Back pain can be felt as a result of (most
likely first):
- sprains (an injury to the ligament of a joint)
- injury (e.g. a car or sporting accident)
- muscle damage (e.g. from over-exercising)
- fractures caused by underlying bone
  disease (e.g. osteoporosis)
- underlying inflammatory disease
  (e.g. rheumatoid arthritis)
- degenerative diseases (e.g. fibromyalgia)
- cancer (e.g. prostate and pancreatic
  cancer)
- infections (e.g. bladder infections and
  spinal infections like tuberculosis).

Simple back pain can be worsened, or
triggered, by a number of factors including:

- poor posture
- a lack of exercise
- standing or bending down for long periods
- sitting in a chair that doesn't provide
  enough back support
- sleeping on an unsuitable mattress
- driving for long periods without a break
- being overweight
- being pregnant
- lifting, carrying, pushing or pulling loads
  that are too heavy.

THE WRONG WAY TO LIFT.

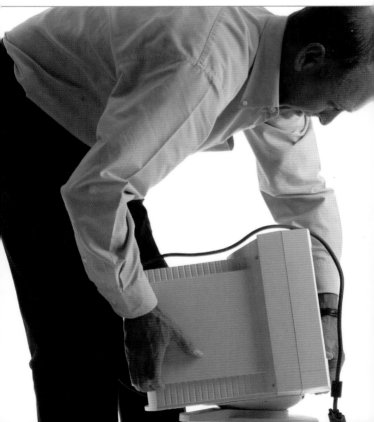

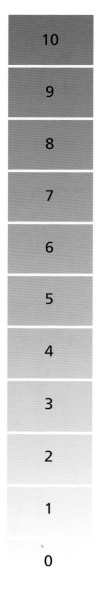

## WHEN SHOULD I SEE A DOCTOR ABOUT MY BACK PAIN?

Most simple back pain gets better on its own after only a few days. Simple painkillers may keep the pain under control (provided they are used as directed on the dosing instructions). However, you should consult your GP if your pain lasts longer than a week or is as a result of a fall or a blow to the back (e.g. a car accident or sporting injury).

You should also consult your doctor if your back pain is accompanied by any of the following symptoms:

- a high temperature
- redness or swelling
- pain down the legs and below the knees
- numbness or weakness in one or both legs
- loss of bladder or bowel control (can indicate pressure on the spinal cord).

## DIAGNOSING BACK PAIN

In the vast majority of cases, your doctor will be able to work out what's wrong by examining you and asking you to describe what your back pain feels like. However, one of the biggest problems with pain is that sometimes we do not have the words to describe it.

Rating pain on a scale of 1 to 10 may help you to describe it more easily.

If your pain lasts longer than it should, or if your doctor suspects that there may be other reasons for your pain, you may be referred for further tests.

## X-rays

■ Shows wear and tear of the spine and broken bones.

## Blood tests

■ Can help to identify very specific causes of pain (e.g. infection, tumours, arthritic diseases).

## CT and MRI scans

■ Provide detailed pictures of bone and surrounding tissues. Can be used to rule out serious diseases.

Even after performing these tests, it may still be unclear why you are in pain. This does not mean that your pain is not genuine or won't be taken seriously, or that nothing can be done to make it easier to live with. Our understanding of pain (and the methods used to bring it under control) has improved dramatically in recent years. For most people, referral to a pain specialist will not be necessary.

## MANAGING BACK PAIN

Healthcare professionals involved in managing your pain will include your GP and may also involve the practice nurse, a pain specialist, a physiotherapist, a counsellor, an occupational health therapist and a pharmacist.

Managing back pain does not just mean taking painkillers or undergoing back surgery. There are many other ways in which you can bring your back pain under control and prevent it from recurring.

Adopting simple changes to your lifestyle can bring about immediate improvements in your back pain. These include:

- staying as active as possible
- losing weight (if you are overweight)
- learning how to bend and lift objects properly
- improving your posture (or adjusting your seating position in the car, at work, at the dinner table, in front of the TV, or your sleeping position).

Contrary to popular opinion, bed rest is not recommended for back pain. It is far better that you try to stay as active as possible. Your doctor will be able to advise you which types of exercise are most suitable.

## ANALGESIA

Painkillers – or analgesics – are drugs that work by interfering with the pain transmission process. Although the stronger analgesics are only available by prescription from your doctor, many of the painkillers that you can obtain over-the-counter from your pharmacist can be effective if taken properly. Remember to always ask your pharmacist for advice and never exceed the stated dose.

## THE DIFFERENT TYPES OF ANALGESIC DRUGS

| Drug | Brand names |
| --- | --- |
| **Over-the-counter (OTC)** | |
| Paracetamol | Calpol®, Disprol®, Hedex®, Panadol® |
| Aspirin | Alka-Seltzer®, Anadin®, Disprin® |
| Ibuprofen | Advil®, Cuprofen®, Nurofen® |
| Compound analgesics: | |
|    Paracetamol and codeine | Solpadeine Max®, Ultramol®, Panadol Ultra® |
|    Aspirin and codeine | Codis 500® |
|    Ibuprofen and codeine | Nurofen® Plus, Solpaflex® |
| **Prescription-only medicines (POM)** | |
| Aspirin | Caprin® |
| Ibuprofen | Arthrofen®, Brufen®, Ebufac®, Motrin® |
| Naproxen | Arthroxen®, Nycopren®, Voltarol® |
| Diclofenac sodium | Acoflam®, Defenac®, Dicloflex®, Volraman® |
| Compound analgesics: | |
|    Paracetamol and codeine | Co-codamol®, Tylex® |
|    Ibuprofen and codeine | Codafen Continus® |
|    Aspirin and codeine | Co-codaprin® |
| Muscle relaxants: | |
|    Diazepam | Rimapam®, Tensium® |
|    Baclofen | Baclospas®, Lioresal® |
| Antiepileptic drugs (for neuropathic pain): | |
|    Carbamazepine | Tegretol® |
|    Gabapentin | Neurontin® |
|    Pregabalin | Lyrica® |
| Opioids: | |
|    Dihydrocodeine | DF 118 Forte®, DHC Continus® |
|    Buprenorphine | Temgesic®, Transtec® |
|    Diamorphine (heroin) | – |
|    Fentanyl | Durogesic®, Actiq® |
|    Morphine | Sevredol®, MST Continus®, Zomorph® |
|    Tramadol | Zydol®, Zamadol® |

*Drugs often have more than one name. A generic name, which refers to its active ingredient, and a brand name, which is the registered trade name given to it by the pharmaceutical company. Ibuprofen is a generic name and Nurofen® is a brand name.*

## THE DOS AND DON'TS OF EFFECTIVELY CONTROLLING BACK PAIN

**1** Don't panic – most spells of back pain will get better.

**2** Don't rest in bed for too long (2–3 days at most).

**3** Do gradually increase your level of activity.

**4** Do back exercises regularly, perhaps take up a new form of exercise (after checking with your doctor).

**5** Do contact your doctor if pain persists for more than a week.

## NON-DRUG TREATMENT

TENS uses small electrical currents to 'block out' pain.

Physiotherapy, osteopathy and chiropractic treatment are all forms of therapy that involve manipulating parts of the backbone to relieve back pain. Transcutaneous Electrical Nerve Stimulation (TENS) and acupuncture can also offer relief from symptoms. Back surgery is rarely necessary and is usually only undertaken as a last resort.

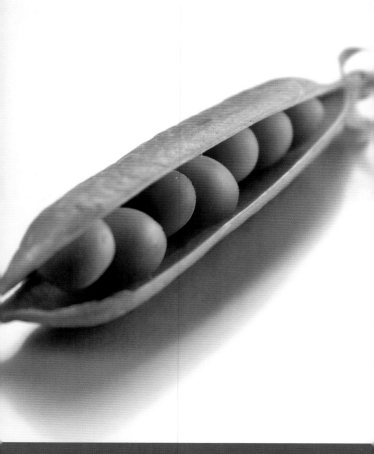

**why me?**

# WHY ME?

If you or someone you know suffers, or has suffered, from back pain, you are by no means alone. Back pain is very common. In the UK, almost half of all adults suffer from back pain that lasts for at least a day each year.

## HOW COMMON IS IT?

In the UK, back pain is the second most common medical complaint, after the common cold.

Back pain is so common that it is highly likely that the majority of us will suffer from it at some point. In the UK, an estimated 60–80% of people are affected by back pain at some time in their lives. Back pain is one of the main reasons for absence from work, and each year millions of working days are lost due to back pain.

In Western countries (e.g. the UK and the USA) the incidence of back pain (particularly pain in the lower back) has reached epidemic proportions. One survey has reported that 17.3 million people in the UK (about one-third of the adult population) are affected by back pain at any one time. Of these, 1.1 million people are disabled by back pain. Low-back pain is the most frequent cause of limitation of activity in the young and middle-aged and is one of the most common reasons for seeking a medical consultation. Every year about 5 million people see their GP because of back pain.

An epidemic is an illness that spreads rapidly through a population or a discrete geographical area.

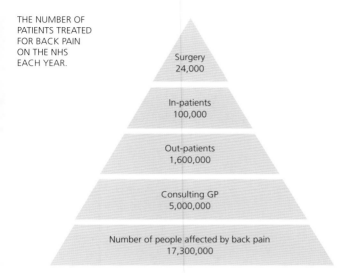

THE NUMBER OF
PATIENTS TREATED
FOR BACK PAIN
ON THE NHS
EACH YEAR.

Surgery
24,000

In-patients
100,000

Out-patients
1,600,000

Consulting GP
5,000,000

Number of people affected by back pain
17,300,000

## CHANGING TRENDS IN BACK PAIN

Back pain is becoming a bigger problem than
it once was. Since the mid-1990s, the
incidence of back pain in the UK has risen by
12.7% and outpatient attendances for back
pain are now five times greater. But why is
this? Many possible explanations have been
proposed:

1  We are more aware of our health and
well-being than we used to be. If we
have a problem we are more likely to
seek medical help than suffer in silence.

2  We expect more from our health
services. When we go to see the doctor
with back pain, we expect them to be
able to do something about it.

**3** We work longer hours than we used to and are under more stress in our everyday lives.

**4** Changes to our diet and the popularity of convenience foods (coupled with our reluctance to exercise) means we are more overweight than we used to be.

**5** We lead increasingly sedentary (or inactive) lifestyles. We drive for longer periods, take less exercise and spend hours sitting in front of the television or computer.

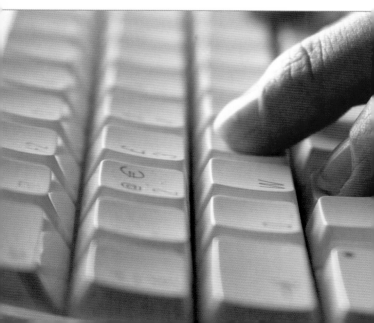

## WHO GETS BACK PAIN?

Whilst we are all at risk of experiencing back pain, some people are more susceptible than others. Back pain becomes more common as we grow older and is most common between the ages of 35 and 55. Even so, children increase their risk of developing back pain by spending too much time hunched over a computer, or by lugging heavy school bags to and from school.

Whether or not (and how frequently) you experience back pain depends on:
- how active you are (your mobility)
- mechanical causes
- underlying diseases
- your job.

Some 30% of children carry school bags that weigh over 10% of their own body weight.

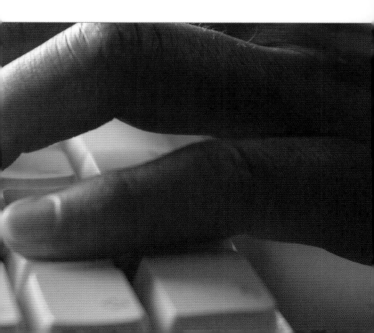

## BACK PAIN AND IMMOBILITY

There are many reasons why we are less active than we used to be. Cars, televisions and computers may make our lives easier, but they are also causing us many health problems. By becoming less active (as well as eating more 'junk' food) we are becoming heavier (and in some cases obese) and our muscles and bones are becoming weaker. These are all risk factors for developing a back complaint.

The UK has the fastest growing prevalence of obesity in the Western world and this is likely to contribute further to back problems in years to come.

Adult obesity rates have almost quadrupled in the last 25 years. Three-quarters of Britons are overweight.

People who are obese have an excessive amount of body fat. A person is considered obese if he or she has a body mass index (BMI) of 30 or greater.

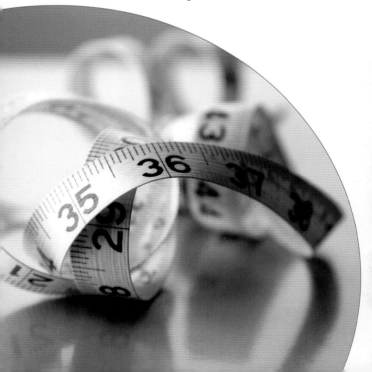

## CALCULATE YOUR OWN BODY MASS INDEX (BMI)

It's very simple to work out your own BMI, to see whether your weight has put you at risk of back pain. Grab a tape measure, a set of bathroom scales and a calculator and follow these two steps.

■ Measure your height in metres. Multiply this number by itself and write down the answer.

■ Measure your weight in kilograms. Divide it by the number you wrote down in the first step. *The number you get is your BMI.*

For example: if your height is 1.80 metres, when you multiply this by itself you get 3.24. If your weight is 80 kilograms, divide 80 by 3.24 to give 24.7.

As a general rule, for adults aged over 20:

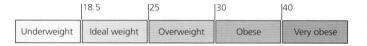

|  | 18.5 | 25 | 30 | 40 |
|---|---|---|---|---|
| Underweight | Ideal weight | Overweight | Obese | Very obese |

Remember though that your BMI is only a broad indicator – it is affected by your body style – people with a very muscular build will have a higher BMI but may not be unhealthily fat. Your age and gender also affect your BMI. Some experts say that men can have a slightly higher BMI before they are at risk, probably due to the fact that they are usually more muscular than women. However, it is best to stick to the guidelines above – they are the internationally accepted boundaries for both genders. The BMI scale does not apply to children though, or during pregnancy.

*Calculate you BMI online at*
*www.bestmedicine.com*

## BACK PAIN AND DRIVING

Our fondness for driving goes hand-in-hand with our tendency to shy away from exercise. Often, we will hop in the car, rather than walk down to the shops or to school or work. Whilst this may save us time, in the long term it may also increase our chances of developing back problems and other health problems. It is well known that people who lead active lifestyles are less likely to die early, or to experience major illnesses such as heart disease, diabetes and colon cancer.

Unfortunately for some people, spending long periods of time sitting in a car is unavoidable (e.g. taxi drivers, bus drivers, salespeople). The constant vibration of the wheels on the road, hunching over or gripping the steering wheel, sitting in the same position and stretching to depress the clutch or see out of the mirror, all take their toll on your back. It's not just the driver who can stiffen up in a car either – passengers are often seated for long periods of time in a fixed position.

If you do spend a lot of time in your car, there are a number of things you can try to make yourself more comfortable:

- bring your seat forward so that you can depress the clutch without having to stretch
- adjust your mirrors properly
- take regular breaks, ideally once an hour
- try to avoid twisting when getting into or out of the car
- keep a small cushion in the car to support your lower back
- choose a car that is suited to your needs.

# CHOOSING THE RIGHT CAR

**The Praying Test** – Place both hands together, pointing forwards. You should be pointing straight at the centre of the steering wheel.

**The Fist Test** – Make a fist with your left hand, keeping the thumb to the side of the index finger. If you have sufficient headroom then it should be possible to insert the fist on the crown of the head.

**The Look Down Test** – Place both hands evenly on the steering wheel and look down at your legs. You should be able to see equal amounts of both legs between the arms.

**The Right Leg Test** – After driving the car for a short while, look down and examine the position of your right leg. Your right foot should still be roughly in line with your right thigh.

**The Kerb Height Test** – Swing your right leg out of the car as though you are getting out, and place your right foot on the ground. The surface of your right thigh should be sloping downwards (not upwards) towards your right knee.

THESE TESTS SHOULD ONLY BE PERFORMED WHEN THE CAR IS STATIONARY AND CAREFULLY PARKED.

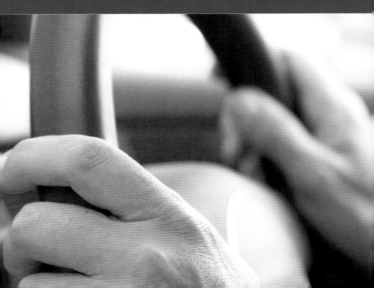

## MECHANICAL CAUSES OF BACK PAIN

Mechanical problems are by far the most common cause of back pain. There are many possible reasons why mechanical pain – in which a specific part of the spine, like a disc, a ligament or a joint, does not work correctly – can occur. As well as strains, knocks and other accidental injuries, a number of diseases can contribute to, or worsen, the mechanical causes of back pain (mentioned in the next section). Remember, underlying disease is not the most common cause of back pain. Some of the mechanics of back pain are discussed below.

### Growing older

Sometimes, back pain is a natural consequence of the ageing process. As we get older the discs that separate the vertebrae lose their flexibility and shock-absorbing properties and are damaged more easily.

### Herniated discs

Although it is often used, the term 'slipped disc' is not strictly accurate. The disc never slips. Instead it usually tears or ruptures and starts to press against nerves from the spinal cord.

This is the process by which one of the discs ruptures and its inner core bulges out through the outer layer of ligaments that surround it. This is painful enough in itself, but if the bulge presses on a spinal nerve, the pain may spread to the part of the body that is served by the nerve. Herniated discs are most common in the lower back and most often affect people between the ages of 25 and 45. Only about 1 in 25 people who have pain in their lower back that is caused by a physical problem have a herniated disc.

A HERNIATED DISC.

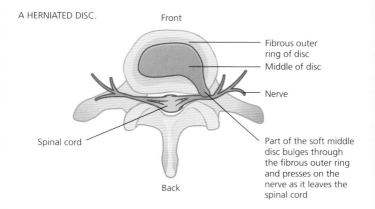

Front

— Fibrous outer ring of disc
— Middle of disc

— Nerve

Spinal cord

Part of the soft middle disc bulges through the fibrous outer ring and presses on the nerve as it leaves the spinal cord

Back

## Facet joint problems

Like the discs, the facet joints that connect the vertebrae together can wear down, or degenerate, and the two halves of the joint can grate against each other, causing back pain.

## Spinal stenosis

Spinal stenosis describes the abnormal narrowing of the spinal canal which then exerts pressure on the spinal cord. Spinal stenosis is usually associated with feelings of weakness or tingling sensations. Another type of stenosis is that of the nerve root canal. This can be linked to the narrowing of the foramina, the space between two vertebrae through which the nerve root passes.

Rheumatoid arthritis comes about when the immune system – the system in the body responsible for fighting diseases and infections – behaves abnormally and starts attacking itself (with antibodies).

One-quarter of all people over the age of 60 have significant pain and disability from arthritis.

## DISEASES THAT CAN CAUSE BACK PAIN

Although they are much less common than the mechanical causes of back pain, certain diseases can contribute to back pain and are likely to need long-term treatment.

### Arthritis

Arthritis is a disease that causes pain in the joints that is usually accompanied by swelling and sometimes changes in their structure. Although arthritis usually affects the knees, ankles and wrists, it can also affect the spine and hip joints, causing chronic back pain. There are two major types of arthritis:

- osteoarthritis – caused by wear and tear of the joints
- rheumatoid arthritis – caused by inflammation in the joints.

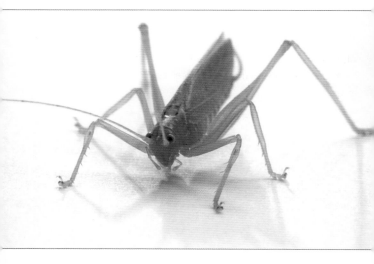

## Ankylosing spondylitis

An extremely rare disease, (affecting about one person in every 1,000) the cause of which is largely unknown. Spondylitis means inflammation of the spine and ankylosing means fusing. The disease is characterised by low-back pain that may spread to the buttocks or thighs but never below the knee. It mainly affects people under the age of 30 and is more common in men than in women.

## Fibromyalgia

A muscle disease that can cause pain all over the body, but mostly affects the neck, spine, shoulders and hips. It can occur as a result of stress, muscle injury or muscle overuse. Fibromyalgia is more common than ankylosing spondylitis and affects between 4 and 20% of people in the UK. People with fibromyalgia often have trouble sleeping.

## Osteoporosis

Although osteoporosis itself does not cause back pain, its long-term consequences can result in significant pain. Vertebral osteoporotic collapse, in which a vertebra breaks down because of underlying osteoporosis, is an example of this.

Osteoporosis is a condition that affects bones and makes them more likely to fracture or break. Our bones are made of a thick outer shell and a strong inner mesh filled with collagen, calcium and other minerals.

Osteoporosis literally means 'porous bones'.

Osteoporosis occurs when the holes in the mesh become bigger, making it more fragile and liable to break easily. Osteoporotic fractures occur most often in the hip, wrist and spine. Spinal fractures are also called vertebral fractures.

Women who have gone through the menopause are particularly susceptible to osteoporosis because they have lower levels of the hormone, oestrogen, which normally slows down the deterioration of bone.

Vertebral fractures can cause back pain, immobility and muscle spasm, to the extent that turning over, sitting up and getting dressed, for example, can become extremely difficult. Interestingly, however, many people with vertebral fractures do not complain of pain and may be unaware that they have a fracture in the first place.

A 50-year-old white woman has a 16% lifetime risk of experiencing a vertebral fracture (compared with 5% in men).

*A detailed scientific review of the available evidence on the drugs used to treat osteoporosis can be found in* BESTMEDICINE Osteoporosis, *available from www.bestmedicine.com*

**FIVE WAYS TO AVOID OSTEOPOROSIS**

- Eat foods rich in calcium
  (e.g. milk, fish, vegetables).

- Eat food rich in vitamin D
  (e.g. oily fish).

- Do regular weight-bearing
  exercise.

- Stop smoking.

- Don't drink too much alcohol.

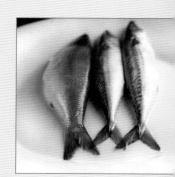

**FIVE WAYS TO AVOID FRACTURES IF YOU HAVE OSTEOPOROSIS**

- Take osteoporosis treatments as
  prescribed by your doctor.

- Fit anti-slip mats around your
  home, especially in the bathroom
  and kitchen.

- Take care when walking on icy or
  slippery surfaces.

- Wear sensible (low-heeled) shoes.

- Make sure your home is well lit.

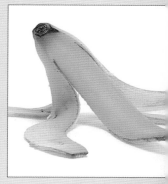

## BACK PAIN AND THE WORKPLACE

Musculoskeletal disorders are diseases that affect the muscles, joints and bones.

Back pain is particularly common in adults who are of a working age. It has been estimated by the Health and Safety Executive (the government body responsible for safety in the workplace) that between 2001 and 2002, millions of working days were lost as a result of musculoskeletal disorders. The majority of these were back pain that was caused or made worse by work. On average, each person with back pain was absent from work for an estimated 18.9 days during this 12-month period. About 13% of unemployed people cite back pain as the reason they are without a job. At any one time, approximately 430,000 people in the UK are receiving Social Security payments for back pain.

Back pain is the second most common cause of sick leave in the world.

## WHICH JOBS ARE MOST OFTEN ASSOCIATED WITH BACK PAIN?

Back pain can arise in many work situations, but certain occupations carry a greater risk then others. These include:

- heavy manual labouring
- heavy equipment operating
- nursing
- delivery work
- removal work
- manual packing of goods
- office work involving sitting at a computer station.

Some 57% of supermarket cashiers report lower back pain within 1 year of starting their jobs.

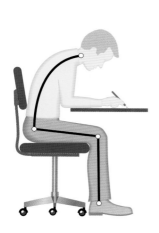 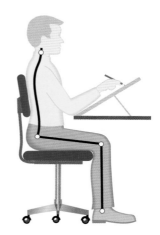

SITTING CORRECTLY (AS IN THE SECOND DIAGRAM) CAN HELP TO PREVENT BACK PAIN.

In general, jobs that involve heavy lifting, handling bulky loads in awkward places, handling vibrating equipment like pneumatic drills or driving long distances over rough ground, can all make back pain worse. Office jobs can also aggravate back pain. Spending all day sitting at a badly adjusted workstation performing a repetitive task like typing or answering the phone, can make the problem worse. A number of exercises can be performed whilst you sit at your desk, which can minimise the chances of suffering from back pain.

## WORK-RELATED TASKS THAT CAN AGGRAVATE BACK PAIN

| Back aggravator | Workers at high risk |
|---|---|
| Lifting heavy objects | Factory workers |
| Lifting awkward or bulky objects | Removal men, nurses |
| Repetitive actions | Typists, telephonists |
| Stretching, twisting, reaching | Mechanics |
| Cold temperatures | Fishermen |
| Vibration | Driller |
| Sitting uncomfortably | Train or bus drivers, supermarket cashiers |

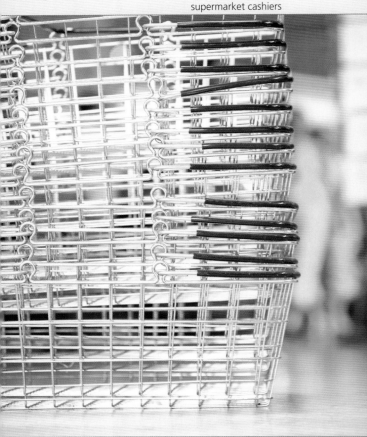

## ERGONOMICALLY SPEAKING

In recent years, we have seen an upsurge in the popularity of specially adapted, 'ergonomic' furniture and equipment, particularly in the workplace. 'Ergonomic' means 'designed for ease of use'. Common examples of ergonomically designed equipment include:

The word 'ergonomic' comes from the Greek words 'ergon' (meaning 'work') and 'nomoi' (meaning 'natural laws').

- chairs designed to prevent the user from sitting in positions that may have a detrimental effect on the spine
- desks with adjustable keyboard trays
- desktops of adjustable heights.

But have the ergonomic improvements we have made to our working conditions made any difference to the incidence of back pain? Although the overall incidence of back pain is increasing for the reasons described previously, there is some evidence to suggest that changes made in the workplace have reduced many serious occupational health risks, including back pain.

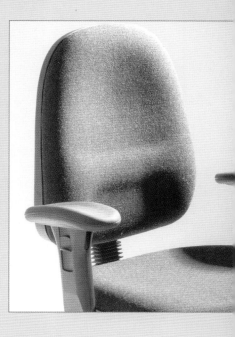

## TEN WAYS TO MAKE YOUR OFFICE MORE ERGONOMICALLY FRIENDLY

1. Make sure you're not stretching for your keyboard and your neck is not bent.
2. Use foot rests and wrist rests if you need to.
3. Keep your feet at right angles to your lower legs.
4. Get your eyes checked regularly so that you are not leaning forward to read your computer screen.
5. Make sure your chair is comfortable and can be adjusted.
6. If possible choose a desk that can be adjusted to the right height for you.
7. Keep your mouse next to and on the same level as your keyboard.
8. Position your keyboard in front of the direction you look to the monitor, not off to the side.
9. Use a telephone headset if you are on the phone constantly.
10. Try not to sit in the same position all day long.

Accidents that take place at work also account for a substantial proportion of back complaints. In the UK, 35% of all reported accidents are due to slips, trips and falls. If you have an accident at work, it is important that you report it using the appropriate channels. Not registering and acting on symptoms quickly enough can sometimes make you feel worse. This may mean recording the incident in an accident report book or obtaining a confirmatory letter from your GP. Your employer or your safety representative will be able to advise you of the accident reporting procedure where you work.

It is your employer's legal responsibility to carry out risk assessments in order to identify possible hazards associated with

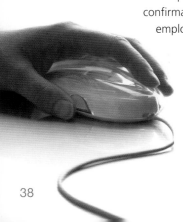

certain jobs. In some cases, using lifting and handling aids can remove or reduce the risk of back injuries. They should accommodate your needs and you should not suffer discrimination as a result of your back problems. You may even be eligible for compensation if you have had an accident at work. For further advice, contact your local Health and Safety Executive (HSE) office (*www.hse.gov.uk*).

Risk assessment is a process that estimates the health risk posed by carrying out a particular task.

1. Lateral head rotation

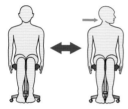

Alternately, turn head 90° to the right and the left, holding for a few moments in each position.

2. Shoulder shrugs

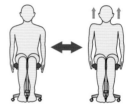

3. Seated calf raises

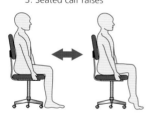

Slowly raise heels upwards and downwards, holding for a few moments each tme.

4. Resisted arm curls

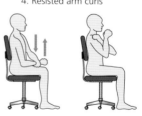

Cross arms. Exerting a downward pressure with the arm on top, raise the lower arm and hold for a few moments.

5. Wrist rolling

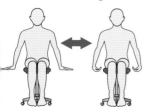

6. Hand/finger exercise

EXERCISES FOR OFFICE WORKERS. 39

# PAIN THROUGH HISTORY

**3000 BC.** The Babylonians believed that people suffering from pain were being punished and frequently enrolled the help of an exorcist and a priest/physician to cure sufferers.

**2600 BC.** The ancient Chinese believed that feeling well was a matter of balancing 'Yin and Yang' (symbols used to illustrate the natural harmony that exists in the world). It was around this time that acupuncture was developed, a treatment that is still used today to manage back pain.

**1550 BC.** In ancient Egypt, pain was believed to be due to the spirits from the dead entering the body through the nostrils or ears. One of the more radical forms of pain relief involved laying electric eels, taken from the Nile, over the wounds of patients.

**1200 BC.** The ancient Greeks argued about whether pain was felt in the heart or the head, although ancient Indians believed that the heart was the root of all pain. It was around this era that opium (the basis of current-day morphine-like painkillers) was first used to relieve pain.

**1400–1500 AD.** Leonardo da Vinci and others of the time were amongst the first to propose that the brain was responsible for sensation and feelings.

**1664 AD.** The French philosopher René Descartes described how particles of fire, in contact with the foot, travel to the brain. He compared pain sensation to the ringing of a bell.

**1800s.** Pain was no longer considered to be a 'gift from God', and was instead seen as a medical challenge.

**1994.** The International Association for the Study of Pain (IASP) defined pain as 'an unpleasant sensory or emotional experience associated with actual or potential tissue damage, or described in terms of such damage'.

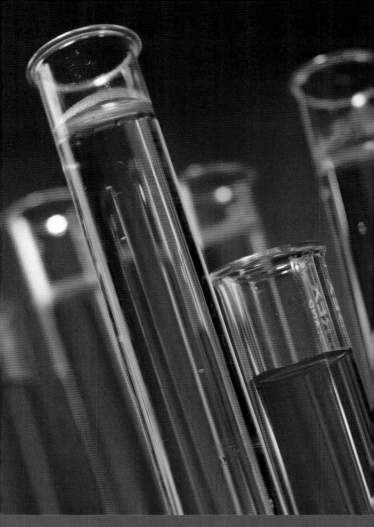

**simple science**

## SIMPLE SCIENCE

Pain transmission (or nociception) is the series of events that takes place in our bodies which allows us to feel and react to pain. It is a very complex process.

## WHEN PAIN HELPS US OUT

1. We are exposed to something that is painful (a painful stimulus). For example, we walk barefoot onto a hot sandy beach.
2. Specialised structures on the soles of our feet called **pain receptors** detect the painful stimulus.
3. The pain receptors send messages to the brain via the spinal cord (time frame – fraction of a second).
4. The brain receives the pain message and interprets it (time frame – fraction of a second).
5. The brain co-ordinates a response to the pain (e.g. get off the beach, run into the sea, put shoes on).

*Pain receptors are located throughout our bodies. Different types of pain receptor detect different types of stimuli (like temperature, pressure and chemicals).*

## WHEN PAIN 'GETS ON OUR NERVES'

Pain becomes a problem to us when it affects the way in which we live our lives (i.e. becomes chronic). For example, if we injure our backs or are suffering from a disease like arthritis, we can experience pain that is persistent. But when does pain become 'a pain'? When our pain machinery becomes sensitised and is activated when it shouldn't be. Pain can be triggered by the irritation of nerve endings (one cause of which is inflammation) or by damage to the nerves.

Pain is generally divided into three types.

■ Acute nociceptive pain usually originates from the site of injury.
■ Inflammatory pain involves the activation of the immune system.
■ Neuropathic pain is usually caused by damage to the peripheral or central nervous systems.

| Type of pain | Cause | How it feels | Examples |
| --- | --- | --- | --- |
| Acute nociceptive | Injury to muscle, soft tissue, bones, joints or skin. | Sharp, stabbing, aching, throbbing. Can be excruciating but is not usually long lasting. | Twisted ankle, bee sting, childbirth. |
| Inflammatory | Generation of inflammatory mediators following a painful stimulus. | Burning, dull ache. Can be excruciating, can come and go, or be virtually permanent. | Rheumatoid arthritis. |
| Neuropathic | Damage to nerve tissue. | Aching, tingling, numbness. Can be excruciating, can come and go, or be virtually permanent. | Trapped or compressed nerve, nerve damage caused by diabetes. |

## HOW DO PAINKILLERS WORK?

All painkillers work by interfering with the pain-transmission process. Although there are many different types, painkillers – or analgesics – usually relieve pain in one of two ways:

■ by predominantly reducing inflammation

or

■ by predominantly affecting the central nervous system.

The central nervous system is made up of the brain and the spinal cord.

## PAINKILLERS THAT ACT BY REDUCING INFLAMMATION

Inflammation is the body's way of responding to injury, infection or invasion by foreign bodies. Inflammation is controlled by **inflammatory mediators**, substances that are made by the body and which may make inflammation worse by sensitising pain receptors.

Prostaglandin, histamine and bradykinin are all pain-causing inflammatory mediators.

Drugs like aspirin and ibuprofen are called non-steroidal anti-inflammatory drugs (NSAIDs). As their name suggests, they work by preventing or limiting inflammation – specifically by blocking the manufacture of prostaglandins. Although prostaglandins do not cause pain themselves, they sensitise nociceptive nerve endings to other inflammatory mediators (like bradykinin and histamine) and thereby amplify the basic pain message.

Prostaglandins are manufactured in the body by an enzyme called cyclo-oxygenase, or 'COX' for short. The COX enzyme helps to

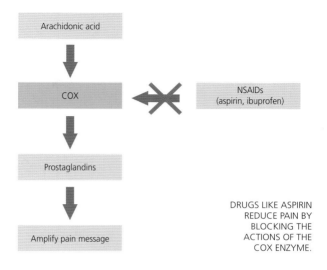

DRUGS LIKE ASPIRIN REDUCE PAIN BY BLOCKING THE ACTIONS OF THE COX ENZYME.

metabolise (or break down) a larger substance called arachidonic acid, into pain-causing prostaglandins.

By attacking COX and stopping it from doing its job properly, aspirin-like drugs slow down the production of the pain-causing prostaglandins. However, slowing down COX is not always a good thing. Confusingly, there are two forms of the COX enzyme – COX-1 and COX-2. Blocking COX-2 ultimately helps to relieve pain. But, most NSAIDs block COX-1 as well, which disrupts other biological processes that are far removed from pain transmission. One of these processes is the production of protective mucus in the stomach. This explains why some people develop gastric ulcers, indigestion and general nausea after taking NSAIDs.

An enzyme is a biological catalyst.

45

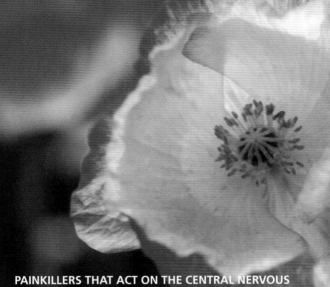

## PAINKILLERS THAT ACT ON THE CENTRAL NERVOUS SYSTEM

The opioids (e.g.morphine and codeine) are the major group of analgesic drugs that work in the brain and spinal cord. These are substances that are derived from the opium poppy and their effects closely resemble those of the endorphins – home-made pain-killing chemicals produced by the body itself.

The effects of the opioids are mediated by opioid receptors, pain-sensing structures which are located both inside and outside the central nervous system. When a drug like morphine acts on an opioid receptor, it blocks the firing of the nerve cell it is attached to, thereby blocking the basic pain message and preventing it from reaching the brain.

Unfortunately, it is very easy to develop tolerance to the pain-relieving effects of opioids. This means that after using these drugs for a prolonged period of time, you will require a larger amount of opioid to give you the same amount of pain relief.

*Put simply, opioids dampen down pain transmission.*

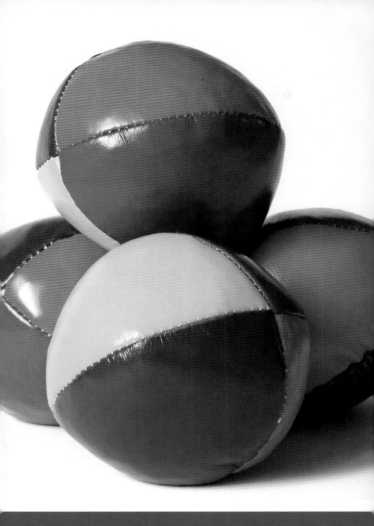

# managing
# back pain

# WHAT MAKES BACK PAIN EASY OR DIFFICULT TO MANAGE?

The degree to which your back pain impinges on your way of living depends on a number of factors:

- how severe your back pain is
- how long it persists
- how active a life you lead
- how old you are.

Mild cases of back pain may mean a couple of days away from work, or that you miss a couple of activities that you had planned. If the pain resolves itself quickly then things will soon return to normal. However, if back pain is severe and/or persists over a long period of time then it may stop you from carrying out your day-to-day activities, lower your self-confidence, disrupt your sleep and in some cases, cause depression.

For the majority of people (90%), back pain will resolve, largely by itself, within 6 weeks or so. Most people (60–70%) end up taking less than a week off work as a result of back pain and 90% of these people are back at work within 2 months. It is when back pain lasts for longer than 3 months that recovery becomes more difficult. In the most extreme cases, some people with chronic back pain never return to work.

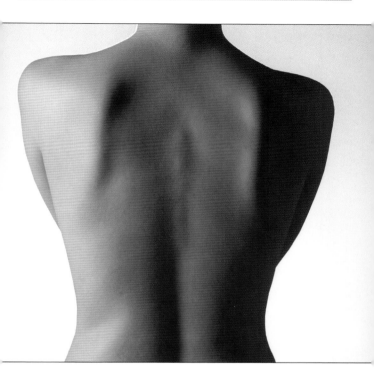

Considering the potentially devastating impact that back pain can have on our lives, it is vital that we are able to recognise and manage it effectively. However, it is important to remember that back pain management means different things to different people. For most of us, mild pain relief and simple changes to our lifestyles are sufficient to make sure that we are able to cope with our pain and to ensure that it doesn't return.

### WHEN SHOULD I SEEK MEDICAL HELP?

Every year about 5 million people see their GP because of back pain.

Many people will be able to manage their back pain without requiring medical advice. Although most back pain usually gets better on its own, within a few days or possibly a few weeks, it is important that you do not suffer in silence. If you become worried about your back pain or it does not seem to be getting any better, then you should make an appointment to see your GP.

In particular, you should consult your GP if your pain lasts longer than a week or is as a result of a fall or a blow to the back (e.g. a car accident or sporting injury). You should also consult your doctor if your back pain is accompanied by any of the following symptoms:

- high temperature
- redness or swelling on the back
- pain down the legs and below the knees
- numbness or weakness in one or both legs
- loss of bladder or bowel control.

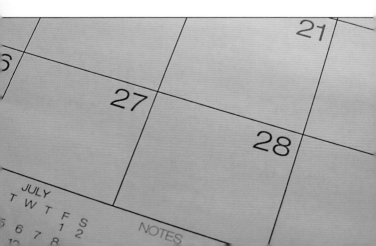

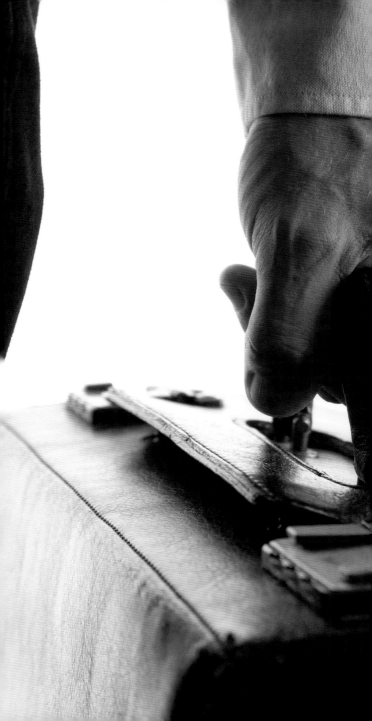

### DIAGNOSING THE CAUSE OF YOUR BACK PAIN

Whilst pain itself does not need to be diagnosed by a doctor, the underlying reason(s) why we experience back pain may be more difficult to pinpoint.

There is no laboratory test that can document the presence or severity of pain.

Pain is very difficult to put into words. In the vast majority of cases, your doctor will try to work out what's wrong with you by asking you to describe what your back pain feels like. It may help you to think about how you would answer the following questions before you visit your doctor.

- Where is your pain?
- Does it stay in the same place?
- What sort of pain is it?
- How long does it last for?
- When did your back pain start?
- What were you doing when it started?
- Have you had any back problems in the past?
- Do you have any other symptoms elsewhere in your body?
- Does your back pain restrict your movement?

To understand how severe pain is, doctors sometimes use a scale of zero (none) to ten (severe) or may ask you to classify the pain as mild, moderate, severe or excruciating. It may

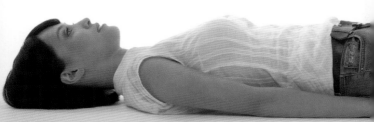

THE STRAIGHT LEG TEST CAN SHOW WHETHER YOU HAVE A DAMAGED DISC.

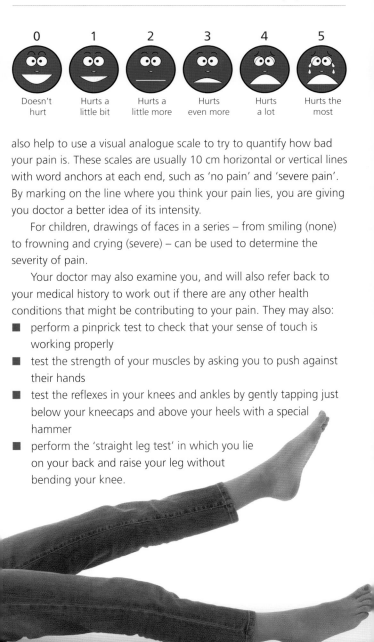

| 0 | 1 | 2 | 3 | 4 | 5 |
|---|---|---|---|---|---|
| Doesn't hurt | Hurts a little bit | Hurts a little more | Hurts even more | Hurts a lot | Hurts the most |

also help to use a visual analogue scale to try to quantify how bad your pain is. These scales are usually 10 cm horizontal or vertical lines with word anchors at each end, such as 'no pain' and 'severe pain'. By marking on the line where you think your pain lies, you are giving you doctor a better idea of its intensity.

For children, drawings of faces in a series – from smiling (none) to frowning and crying (severe) – can be used to determine the severity of pain.

Your doctor may also examine you, and will also refer back to your medical history to work out if there are any other health conditions that might be contributing to your pain. They may also:

■ perform a pinprick test to check that your sense of touch is working properly

■ test the strength of your muscles by asking you to push against their hands

■ test the reflexes in your knees and ankles by gently tapping just below your kneecaps and above your heels with a special hammer

■ perform the 'straight leg test' in which you lie on your back and raise your leg without bending your knee.

## 'RED FLAGS'

There are a number of signs and symptoms that will alert your doctor to a specific cause of pain, so-called 'red flags'. These include:

- your age (if you are younger than 20 or older than 55)
- whether you have sustained a serious injury (e.g. road accident)
- pain that is getting worse
- pain in the upper part of your spine
- you have, or have had, cancer
- you are taking steroids
- you have HIV
- you are a recreational drug user
- you have lost a lot of weight
- you are experiencing numbness or significant weakness.

Rarely, your GP may be unable to find the cause of the pain and may refer you for further tests (including X-rays, computed tomography [CT] and magnetic resonance imaging [MRI] scans). These tests are not usually painful themselves, and won't take very long to carry out. They will usually take place in a hospital or a specialist pain clinic.

### CT and MRI scans

CT and MRI scans are relatively quick and easy ways of obtaining detailed images of the inside of the body, without needing to perform surgery.

During a CT scan, X-rays are passed through the body at various angles. As they leave the body, the X-rays are detected by a scanner which uses the information to produce a two-dimensional image of the internal structures of the back. CT scanners are increasingly being replaced by MRI scanners, which use radiowaves (which are safer than X-rays) and high-powered magnetic fields to create two- or three-dimensional images. MRI scanners can distinguish between bone and soft tissue and therefore provide a more detailed picture of the inside of the body.

## Myelography and discography

Patients undergoing myelography have a coloured dye injected into their spinal canal and are then tipped up and down on an X-ray table whilst radiographic images are taken. Although these days myelography is not so risky, in the past, some patients experienced arachnoiditis – painful inflammation of the spinal cord – after they were injected with the dye Myodil®.

In discography the dye is injected into the disc that separates one vertebra from the next. This outlines the damaged area of the disc and can help to pinpoint the cause of the pain.

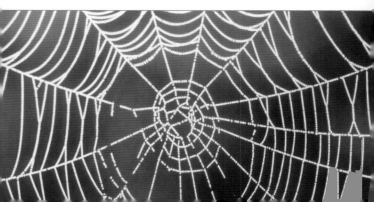

## DIAGNOSTIC TESTS USED TO DETERMINE THE CAUSES OF BACK PAIN

| Test | Advantages |
|------|------------|
| X-ray | • Can usually rule out any serious diseases.<br>• Shows wear and tear of the spine and broken bones.<br>• Quick and painless. |
| Blood tests | • Can be used to determine very specific causes of pain (e.g. infection, tumours, arthritic diseases). |
| CT scanning | • Quick and painless.<br>• Can be used to rule out serious diseases. |
| MRI scanning | • The most advanced type of scan.<br>• Quick and painless.<br>• Gives high quality images of bone and surrounding tissues.<br>• Can be used to rule out serious diseases.<br>• Radiowaves are 'safer' than X-rays. |
| Myelography | • Can pinpoint exact causes of back pain. |
| Discography | • Can pinpoint exact causes of back pain. |

*Even after performing these tests, it may still be unclear why you are in pain. This does not mean that nothing can be done to ease the pain and make it easier to live with.*

## Disadvantages

- Will not show up nerve problems.
- Cannot be used alone to determine the cause of pain.
- Exposure to too many X-rays can be dangerous.

- Only detect very specific causes of pain.
- Results must be confirmed by other tests.

- Increasingly replaced by MRI scanning.
- Exposure to too many X-rays can be dangerous.
- Waiting lists can be long.

- Injection of dye can be uncomfortable.
- More complicated than CT and MRI scans.
- Exposure to too many X-rays can be dangerous.
- Arachnoiditis (painful inflammation of the spinal cord) is a rare side-effect.

- Injection of dye can be uncomfortable.
- More complicated than CT and MRI scans.
- Exposure to too many X-rays can be dangerous.

*Your doctor – in consultation with their colleagues and most importantly with you – will be able to put together a personal pain management plan to help you to control your pain.*

### YOUR BACK PAIN MANAGEMENT PLAN

It is important that you work with your GP to formulate a pain management plan that is tailored to suit your individual needs. According to guidelines set out by the NHS, any back pain management plan should aim to:

- relieve your pain symptoms
- help you to recover from acute attacks of pain within 6 weeks
- minimise the amount of time you spend off work
- allow you to resume your normal level of activity
- prevent episodes of acute low-back pain from recurring and becoming chronic problems
- effectively manage back pain if it does become chronic.

Over the course of your back pain management, you may come into contact with a number of different healthcare professionals. Quite often, people with chronic pain are seen by a combination of doctors, nurses, physiotherapists, pharmacists, psychologists and occupational therapists, who offer their expertise and help them to deal with their pain.

Your pain management team will include your GP and may include the practice nurse, a pain specialist, a physiotherapist, a counsellor, an occupational health therapist and a pharmacist.

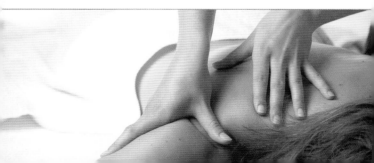

As well as receiving treatment on a one-to-one basis, some people with chronic pain may be able to attend specialist pain clinics for treatment and advice on living a fuller life in spite of their pain. Some healthcare teams may bring together groups of patients with similar pain problems and look at how best to tackle them. Pain services may vary from area to area. Your GP will be able to put you in touch with local support groups and services (see Simple Extras).

## WILL I BE REFERRED?

For the vast majority of people with back pain, a referral to a specialist is not necessary. However, for some people, referral may help to confirm, establish or exclude a diagnosis. Rarely, it may be appropriate for a specialist to arrange or undertake a surgical treatment procedure.

Referral may be appropriate if:

- nerve root pain has not resolved after 4 weeks
- sciatica has not resolved after 6 weeks
- there are other symptoms such as bowel and bladder problems
- feelings of weakness or numbness are getting worse
- your GP suspects you may have an inflamed spine
- you haven't got back to normal within 3 months.

You experience back pain that is persistent

You consult your GP who makes a diagnosis

You and your GP discuss the options and agree a personal pain management plan

Your pain is brought under control

## LIFESTYLE CHANGES

After 12 months, 9 out of 10 people who stayed active during their pain were back at work. Only 5 out of 10 people who did not stay active had resumed work by this time.

Before, or indeed as well as, using drug treatment to alleviate pain, there are a number of lifestyle changes you can make that may improve your back pain. These include:

- staying as active as possible
- losing weight
- learning how to bend and lift objects properly
- improving your posture
- avoiding bed rest.

The number one misconception surrounding back pain is that putting your feet up or staying in bed will help you to get better. In fact the reverse is probably true – bed rest may slow down your recovery. Medical evidence has shown that staying in bed for 2 to 7 days is worse than a placebo or ordinary activity.

A placebo is an inactive substance which may look like a medicine but has no medicinal value.

If you are able to, staying active is one of the best things you can do to relieve back pain. This is because it maintains your muscle strength, fitness and flexibility and speeds up your rehabilitation, helping you to resume your normal way of living more quickly. You should consult your doctor before taking up any new form of exercise and always remember to warm up properly before exercising.

### WHY IS BED REST BAD FOR YOUR BACK?

- It stiffens your joints.
- It weakens your muscles.
- It can weaken your bones over long periods.

## TOP TIPS FOR A 'BACK-FRIENDLY' BED

- Choose a mattress that is supportive enough to take the weight of your body without sagging.
- Turn your mattress regularly (every 6 to 12 weeks).
- Choose a mattress that is comfortable to lie on with sufficient 'give' to cushion your bony bits.
- Buy a mattress with a strong base. Always try out the mattress and base together in the shop before buying.
- Consider a water bed – they support the body without distorting the spine, and are popular with some people.

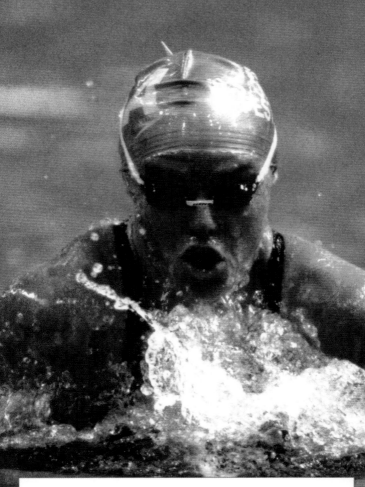

Sports that can **help to relieve** back pain:

- gentle exercises
- walking
- cycling
- swimming (very good because it strengthens muscles whilst supporting the body with water).

Sports which are **not very good** for back pain:

- jogging
- football
- golf
- ballet/gymnastics
- weight lifting.

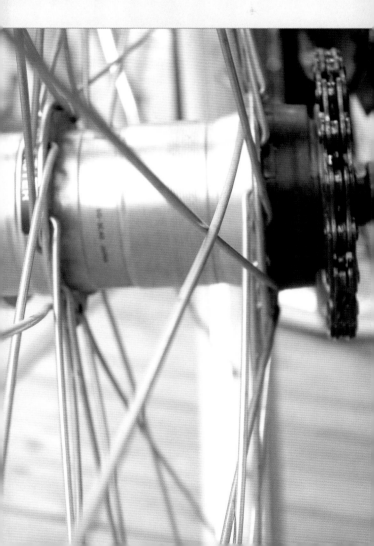

# STRETCHING EXERCISES FOR BACK PAIN

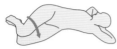

NB: Upper knee should be directly above lower knee

### 1. Back stretch
Lie on your back with your knees bent. Keeping your feet on the floor, slowly roll your knees over, first to one side and then the other, holding for a few seconds in each position.

### 3. One-leg stand – front
Using a wall for support, bend your leg behind you as shown (holding for a few moments each time).

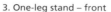
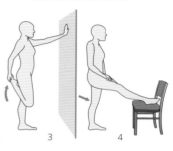

### 4. One-leg stand – back
Placing one leg on a chair as shown, bend your supporting knee to stretch the hamstrings out.

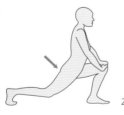

### 2. Deep lunge
Whilst kneeling on one knee in a forward-facing position, slowly lift the other knee upwards, holding for a few seconds each time.

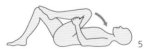

### 5. Knee to chest
Lying on your back, bend one leg and gently hug it to your chest for a few moments.

# BENDING EXERCISES FOR BACK PAIN

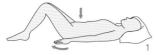

### 1. Pelvic tilt
Whilst lying on your back with your knees bent, use your stomach muscles to flatten your back against the floor, holding for a few seconds each time.

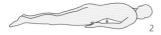

### 2. Stomach tone
Whilst lying on your front with your head to one side, tighten your stomach muscles, holding for a few seconds each time. This exercise can also be performed whilst you are sitting or standing.

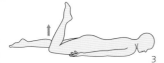

### 3. Buttock tone
Whilst lying on your front, bend one leg upwards and lift your bent knee just off the floor, holding for a few seconds each time.

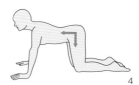

### 4. Deep stomach muscle tone
Kneeling on all fours, relax your stomach completely. Next, move the lower part of your stomach upwards so that your back is lifted away from the floor (without arching).

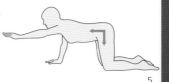

### 5. Back stabiliser
Whilst kneeling on all fours with your back straight, extend one arm out in front of you, holding for a few moments. Repeat with the other arm and ultimately, lift your leg out behind you instead.

Where appropriate, repeat exercises for the same number of times on each side.

## THE DRUG MANAGEMENT OF BACK PAIN

Painkillers – or analgesics – are drugs that work by interfering with the pain transmission process.

Depending on the cause and type of your back pain, some analgesics may be more appropriate then others. Paracetamol and aspirin-like drugs (non-steroidal anti-inflammatory drugs [NSAIDs]) are often used to relieve pain caused by musculoskeletal conditions, whereas the opioid analgesics, codeine and morphine, are more suitable for treating moderate or severe pain that originates from damage to the internal organs of the body (e.g. the heart, lungs, liver, bladder, kidney and reproductive organs).

The appropriateness of the various types of drugs also depends on whether your pain is acute or chronic. Although many of the drugs used are the same, they may be used at different doses or more or less frequently.

Whilst your doctor can prescribe you a number of different types of painkiller, in many cases, drugs that can be purchased without a prescription are sufficient to relieve many kinds of back pain. You can buy these drugs yourself from your pharmacist, and if you pay for your prescriptions, this may be cheaper than acquiring the same drug from your doctor with a prescription. Your pharmacist will advise you which types of drug are most appropriate for you. Always take medication as directed on the packaging and consult your doctor if the pain persists.

Acute pain lasts for less than 8 weeks and chronic pain generally lasts for more than 2 months.

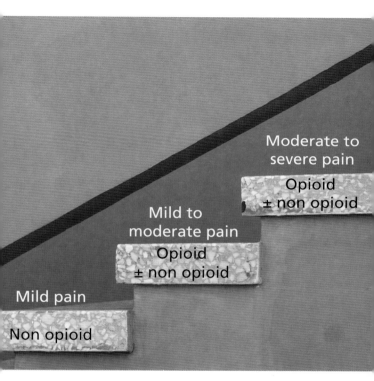

Moderate to
severe pain

Opioid
± non opioid

Mild to
moderate pain

Opioid
± non opioid

Mild pain

Non opioid

PAIN RELIEF IS
USUALLY A STEP-BY-
STEP PROCESS
(WHO).

Since some types of analgesic are stronger than others, you will usually start with one of the weaker drugs and if this fails to relieve your pain sufficiently, you may work your way up to a stronger drug. If the stages in pain relief are considered to be like the rungs of a ladder, then most people will have their pain relieved at the lowest rung. The higher up the pain relief ladder you go, the more likely you are to experience unpleasant drug-related side-effects.

## THE DRUG DEVELOPMENT PROCESS

Developing and launching a new drug onto the commercial market is an extremely costly and time-consuming venture. The process can take a pharmaceutical company between 10 and 15 years from the outset, at an estimated cost of £500 million. Much of this time is spent fulfilling strict guidelines set out by regulatory authorities in order to ensure the safety and quality of the end product. Once registered, a new drug is protected by a patent for 20 years, after which time other rival companies are free to manufacture and market identical drugs, called generics. Thus, the pharmaceutical company has a finite period of time before patent expiry to recoup the costs of drug development and return a profit to their shareholders.

During the development process, a drug undergoes five distinct phases of rigorous testing – the preclinical phase, which takes place in the laboratory – and phases 1, 2, 3 and 4, which involve testing in humans. Approval from the regulatory body and hence, a licence to sell the drug, is dependent on the satisfactory completion of all phases of testing. In the UK, the Medicines and Healthcare Products Regulatory Agency (MHRA) and the European Medicines Evaluation Agency (EMEA) regulate the drug development process.

- Only about 1 in every 100 drugs that enter the preclinical stage progress into human testing because they failed to work or had unacceptable side-effects.
- Animal testing is an important part of drug development. Before a drug reaches a human, it is vital that its basic safety has been established in an animal. Researchers do everything in their powers to minimise the number of animals they use and must adhere to strict guidelines issued by the Home Office.
- Phase 1 testing takes place in groups of 10–80 healthy volunteers.
- Phase 2 testing takes place in 100–300 patients diagnosed with the disease the drug is designed to treat.
- Phase 3 clinical trials involve between 1,000 and 3,000 patients with the relevant disease, and look at both the short- and long-term effects of the drug.
- Phase 4 testing and monitoring continues after the drug has reached the market.

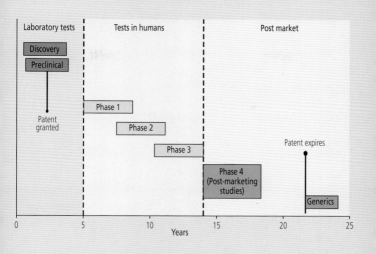

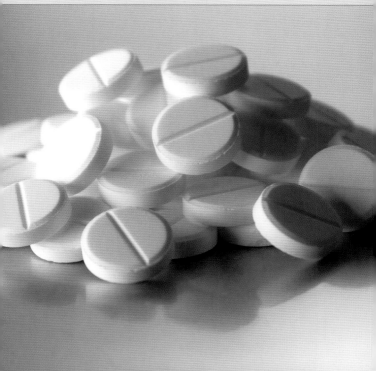

## ANALGESIC DRUGS AVAILABLE OVER-THE-COUNTER (OTC)

| Drug name | Brand names |
|---|---|
| Paracetamol | Calpol®, Disprol®, Hedex®, Panadol® |
| **NSAIDs** | |
| Aspirin | Alka-Seltzer®, Anadin®, Disprin® |
| Ibuprofen | Advil®, Cuprofen®, Nurofen® |
| **Compound analgesics** | |
| Paracetamol and codeine | Solpadeine Max®, Ultramol®, Panadol Ultra® |
| Aspirin and codeine | Codis 500® |
| Ibuprofen and codeine | Nurofen® Plus, Solpaflex® |
| Paracetamol and dihydrocodeine | Paramol® |

## ANALGESIC DRUGS ONLY AVAILABLE WITH A PRESCRIPTION (POM)

| Drug name | Brand names |
|---|---|
| **NSAIDS** | |
| Aspirin | Caprin® |
| Ibuprofen | Arthrofen®, Brufen®, Ebufac®, Motrin® |
| Naproxen | Arthroxen®, Nycopren®, Voltarol® |
| Diclofenac sodium | Acoflam®, Defenac®, Dicloflex®, Volraman® |
| Indometacin | Rimacid®, Indomax 75 SR®, Indomod® |
| **Compound analgesics** | |
| Paracetamol and codeine | Co-codamol®, Tylex® |
| Ibuprofen and codeine | Codafen Continus® |
| Aspirin and codeine | Co-codaprin® |
| **Muscle relaxants** | |
| Diazepam | Rimapam®, Tensium® |
| Baclofen | Baclospas®, Lioresal® |
| **Antiepileptic drugs** | |
| Carbamazepine | Tegretol® |
| Gabapentin | Neurontin® |
| Pregabalin | Lyrica® |
| **Opioids** | |
| Dihydrocodeine | DF 118 Forte®, DHC Continus® |
| Buprenorphine | Temgesic®, Transtec® |
| Diamorphine (heroin) | – |
| Fentanyl | Durogesic®, Actiq® |
| Morphine | Sevredol®, MST Continus®, Zomorph® |
| Tramadol | Zydol®, Zamadol® |

**Over-the-counter painkillers (OTC)**

- paracetamol
- non-steroidal anti-inflammatory drugs (NSAIDs) ['aspirin-like' drugs]
- compound analgesics (e.g. paracetamol plus codeine).

**Prescription-only medicines (POM)**

- stronger doses of NSAIDs
- stronger doses of compound analgesics
- muscle relaxants
- antiepileptic drugs (for neuropathic pain only)
- opioids.

### Paracetamol

Paracetamol and aspirin-like drugs are generally equally effective at relieving pain, but paracetamol is less irritating to the stomach. For this reason, it is often used preferentially in the elderly and in other susceptible groups of people like pregnant women, those with asthma and those with gastric ulcers. Overdosing on paracetamol is extremely dangerous because it may cause permanent and irreversible damage to your liver. Always take paracetamol as directed on the packaging (two 500 mg tablets every 4 hours up to a maximum of eight tablets in 24 hours) and consult your doctor if your pain persists. You should also be aware that paracetamol can be 'hidden' in some branded products and take extra care not to overdose inadvertently.

PARACETAMOL CAN BE 'HIDDEN' IN SOME BRANDED PRODUCTS.

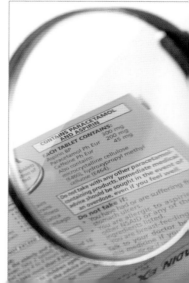

## Non-steroidal anti-inflammatory drugs (NSAIDs)

Aspirin was introduced onto the drug market in 1899, and within a few years, it had become one of the most popular drugs on Earth.

NSAIDs like aspirin and ibuprofen are amongst the most widely used types of pain relief. Aspirin is also widely used to prevent the formation of blood clots in people who are at risk of developing cardiovascular disease. Because, like paracetamol, they start to work quickly, NSAIDs are often used to relieve acute pain. The major problem associated with NSAIDs is the irritation they cause to the stomach and digestive system. Taking these drugs after eating can help to prevent this. NSAIDs are not suitable for:

- people over 65 years of age
- people with a history of gastric ulcers
- people using blood-thinning drugs like warfarin
- people with some other diseases like heart disease, kidney disease, diabetes and asthma.

### The cyclo-oxygenase-2 (COX-2) inhibitors

The COX-2 inhibitors (e.g. celecoxib [Celebrex®], etodolac [Eccoxolac®], etoricoxib [Arcoxia®] and meloxicam [Mobic®] are NSAIDs that are used to relieve the joint (and back) pain associated with arthritis. In contrast to other NSAIDs, these drugs do not disrupt the stomach and digestive systems so much and this is seen as a major advantage for those people who have to take them on a regular basis.

Recently, evidence has emerged to suggest that some types of COX-2 inhibitors (e.g. rofecoxib [Vioxx®] and celecoxib [Celebrex®] may increase the likelihood of cardiovascular complications (like heart attacks) in some people. Therefore, as a precaution, it is recommended that these drugs should only be used in people who are particularly susceptible to the gastrointestinal side-effects of standard NSAIDs, and only after their risk of heart complications has been measured and found to be low. If you are currently taking any of these drugs and have concerns, you should contact your GP.

More recent evidence suggests that not just the COX-2 inhibitors but all NSAIDs (including ibuprofen and naproxen) can be linked to an increased risk of having a heart attack. It should be emphasised that this is only preliminary data and further investigation into these drugs is needed before any firm conclusions can be reached. In the meantime, try to use the lowest effective dose of NSAID for the shortest time necessary.

### Compound analgesics

Compound analgesics are tablets that contain both a simple analgesic (such as aspirin or paracetamol) and a low dose of an opioid analgesic (such as codeine). Solpadeine®, Solpaflex® and Co-Codamol® are all examples of compound analgesics. Depending on how strong they are, these drugs can be obtained either over-the-counter or as prescription-only medicines that you must be given by your doctor.

Co-proxamol®, a compound analgesic containing paracetamol and dextropropoxyphene, was until recently used by many people suffering from the chronic pain associated with arthritis. However, from 2005 Co-proxamol® is being withdrawn from general use because of concerns that it is too dangerous if taken in large quantities.

### Muscle relaxants

Although not strictly analgesic drugs, muscle relaxants like diazepam (Rimapam®, Tensium®) and baclofen (Baclospas®, Lioresal®) can relieve back pain by relaxing muscle spasm and thereby allowing you to be more active. Although diazepam is the most widely used drug for this purpose, there is a slight risk of becoming physically dependent (addicted) if you use it for longer than 2 weeks. Diazepam can also cause drowsiness. For this reason, this type of drug is usually only given to people with back pain who suffer from severe episodes of muscle spasm.

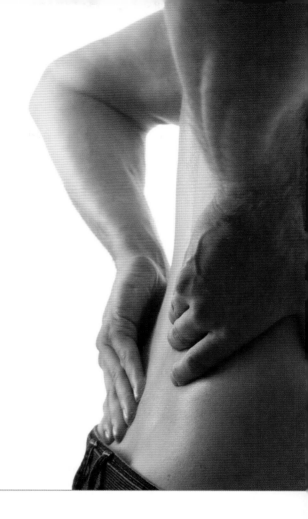

### Antiepileptic drugs

Also known as anticonvulsants, antiepileptic drugs like carbamazepine (Tegretol®), gabapentin (Neurontin®) and pregabalin (Lyrica®) can sometimes be used to treat certain types of neuropathic pain. The exact way in which these drugs relieve pain is not fully understood.

### Opioid analgesics

Opioids – medications derived from the opium poppy – have been used in pain management for hundreds of years. Currently, more than 20 different opioids are available in the UK. Most of these are taken as tablets, but opioids can also be injected or delivered via a patch applied to the skin. Opioids can be divided into 'weak' and 'strong' categories. This classification may be slightly misleading, because in fact no opioid is a 'weak' drug, and all should be taken with extreme care.

People who are addicted to opioids feel a compelling need to take them, even though they may be interfering with their physical or mental well-being.

If your back pain is particularly severe or persistent than your doctor may prescribe you a short course of strong opioids (e.g fentanyl,

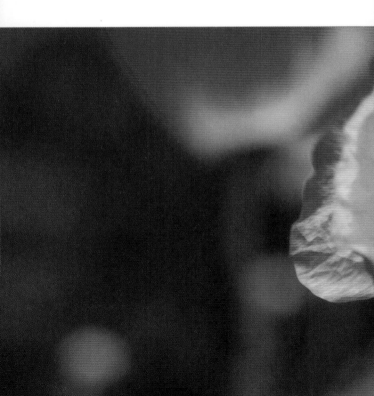

morphine), although these drugs are often used as a last resort because they are associated with a number of unpleasant side-effects. You should not drink alcohol when you are taking opioids, and whilst your dose of opioid is being adjusted it is not advisable that you drive a car.

If opioids are not taken according to the directions of your doctor, they can sometimes cause severe breathing difficulties. Addiction to opioids is extremely rare in people who are taking opioids to treat pain and is instead more likely to affect those people who abuse these drugs recreationally.

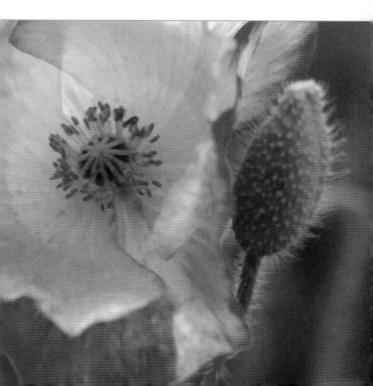

### Off-licence indications

Before they can be used in people, all drugs must be granted a licence. The licence will set out exactly which diseases and conditions the drug can legally be used to treat. Any medicinal use of the drug that is not covered in the terms of the licence is called an 'off-licence indication'. Your doctor may prescribe you a drug for an off-licence indication but this is done at their discretion.

Currently, antidepressants (like amitryptiline [Triptafen®]) are not licensed for pain control in the UK. However, there is strong evidence from clinical trials that some types of these drugs can help to relieve pain by brightening a person's mood and dulling the pain signals being sent to their brain. Your doctor may feel that your pain may respond well to antidepressants and may prescribe you a course of treatment.

Another example of an off-licence indication is the injection of corticosteroids into the epidural space in the back. This is rather an extreme measure because it eliminates the sensation of pain from the waist downwards, and it is therefore usually reserved for extreme cases of back pain. People with severe sciatica may benefit from epidural pain relief. Epidural steroids are usually injected by anaesthetists or other medical specialists in a hospital setting.

The doses of antidepressants that are used to relieve pain are much lower than those used to treat people with depression.

The epidural space is the area between the nerves of the spinal cord and the lining surrounding them.

## THE SIDE-EFFECTS OF DRUG TREATMENT

No drug treatment is without its side-effects. People may respond in slightly different ways to the same medicine. If you experience symptoms which you think may be due to the medication you are taking, you should talk to your doctor, pharmacist or nurse. If the side-effect is unusual or severe, your GP may decide to report it to the MHRA. The MHRA operates a 'Yellow Card Scheme' which is designed to flag up potentially dangerous drug effects and thereby protect your safety. The procedure has changed recently to allow patients to report adverse drug reactions themselves. Visit *www.yellowcard.gov.uk* for more information.

> **You should always ask your doctor if you are concerned about any aspect of your pain management.**

'MHRA' stands for the Medicines and Healthcare Products Regulatory Agency.

### THE SIDE-EFFECTS MOST FREQUENTLY ASSOCIATED WITH ANALGESIC DRUGS

| Drug type | Side-effects |
| --- | --- |
| Paracetamol | Rashes, liver problems (rarely). |
| NSAIDs | Abdominal pain, diarrhoea, swelling. |
| Compound analgesics | A combination of the side-effects associated with each individual component. |
| Muscle relaxants | Drowsiness, lightheadedness, confusion, physical dependence, muscle weakness, forgetfulness, difficulty speaking, agitation. |
| Antiepileptic drugs | Diarrhoea, dry mouth, nausea, vomiting, dizziness, drowsiness, anxiety, amnesia, tremor, constipation, confusion, weight gain, visual disturbances. |
| Opioids | Nausea, vomiting, itching, drowsiness, constipation. |
| Antidepressants | Dry mouth, drowsiness, blurred vision, constipation, nausea, rapid pulse, sweating, tremor. |
| Epidural injection of steroids | Discomfort on injection. |

## THE PHYSICAL TREATMENT OF BACK PAIN

Physiotherapy, osteopathy and chiropractic treatment can all help to relieve back pain. All of these techniques involve manipulating parts of the backbone and some can involve exercise, massage and ultrasound therapy. All must be carried out by a suitably qualified professional. By correcting any underlying mechanical disturbances in the musculoskeletal system, manipulation can effectively relieve the pain and distress of back pain and minimise the need for drug treatment and the risks associated with this. However, manipulation is not recommended in some people, including pregnant women and people with osteoarthritis of the neck or osteoporosis of the spine. If manipulation is inappropriate for you then your GP will let you know.

It is important that you choose a physiotherapist, osteopath or a chiropractor who is suitably qualified. There are a number of regulatory bodies in place to help you do this. By choosing a therapist who is registered with the Chartered Society of Physiotherapy (*www.csp.org.uk*), the General Osteopathic Council (*www.osteopathy.org.uk*) or the General Chiropractic Council (*www.gcc-uk.org*), you are automatically ensuring that you receive the best standard of care.

The first time you visit a therapist they will take a full medical history and ask you about your general health, lifestyle, emotional state and family history. This may take an hour or so. Subsequent consultations will usually last about half an hour.

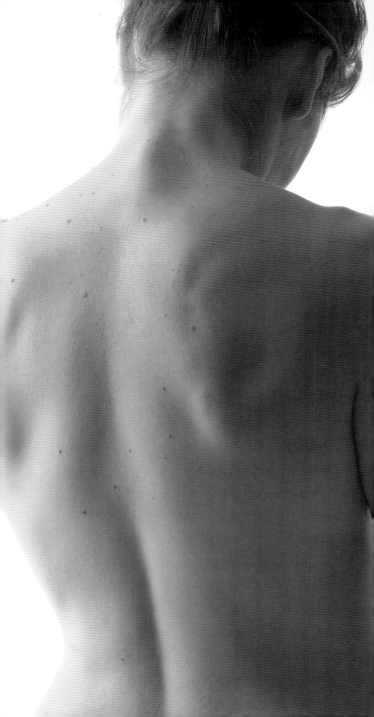

### Going private

Whilst it is possible that your GP may refer you for manipulation, a referral is not essential. There is no need to apologise to your doctor for seeing a physiotherapist, osteopath or chiropractor independently, but it is a good idea to keep them informed of exactly what other treatments you are receiving. Whether you see these practitioners privately or through the NHS, the standard of care you will receive is exactly the same. However, if you are willing to pay for the treatment yourself, it may be that you get seen faster than you would if you waited to go through the NHS.[1] If you choose to approach a practitioner directly and pay for your treatment, fees range from £25 to £50 for a single session. It may also be possible to claim for your treatment if you have a private health insurance policy.

### Physiotherapy

Physiotherapy uses physical means (such as massage, exercise, heat or electricity) to maintain and restore your physical and mental well-being. It is an active rather than a passive treatment and is usually concerned with keeping your joints and muscles moving. As well as relieving back pain, physiotherapy can also be used to treat a large number of other common ailments like muscle sprains, sports

---

[1]In some areas, osteopathy and chiropractic treatment is not available under the NHS.

injuries, incontinence, osteoporosis, depression and asthma. Physiotherapy is heavily based on the basic principles of medical science, and is therefore generally regarded as a conventional rather than a complementary kind of therapy. Physiotherapists work in all areas of the NHS, private healthcare, industry and education, and physiotherapy is the fourth largest healthcare profession in the country.

Osteopathy was developed in the late nineteenth century by an American called Andrew Taylor Still.

# OSTEOPATHY

*Osteopathy uses the manipulation of the body and the spine to cure disease. Over half of people who go to an osteopath do so for back pain. Osteopaths use their hands and fingers to feel the patient's body and identify damaged areas. These areas may have a slightly different temperature or tone, or respond differently to movement than normal healthy areas of the body. Once the injured area has been found, a variety of manual techniques are used to try to correct the problem. Osteopathy usually also involves a special form of massage that helps muscles relax and lets joints move more easily. Osteopathy is not recommended for some people with back pain, including people with brittle bone conditions or inflamed joints, and women in the early stages of pregnancy.*

# CHIROPRACTIC TREATMENT

*Like osteopaths, chiropractors aim to diagnose and correct joint disorders. Although at first glance the two techniques may appear to be very similar, they are in fact quite different. Osteopathy uses more soft tissue massage and osteopaths suggest that the benefits of their therapy are related to the improved circulation of the blood. In contrast, chiropractors suggest that their treatment improves nervous function and relieves pain in this way. Around half of all chiropractic consultations are for low-back pain, including hip problems. The technique was developed in the late nineteenth century by a Canadian called Daniel David Palmer.*

*After examining you, chiropractors are able to identify whether the contraction of the muscles surrounding the spinal column has pulled the spine out of line slightly, and is thus causing your pain. Once it has been identified, chiropractors try to rectify the problem by reducing the tension in these muscles so that the spinal column becomes straighter and exerts less pressure on your joints, thereby lessening your pain. Chiropractic treatment is not suitable for people with inflamed joints, spinal infections or cancer. Treatment can be specially adapted to suit those people with osteoporosis or fractures.*

'Chiropractic' comes from the Greek 'cherio' and 'praktikos' and means 'done by hand'.

## ALTERNATIVE WAYS TO MANAGE BACK PAIN

### Transcutaneous Electrical Nerve Stimulation (TENS)

TENS is a type of pain relief that is centred around using small electrical currents to 'block out' the nerves that are transmitting the feelings of pain you are experiencing. Instead of pain, you will feel more tolerable tingling sensations. Small pads are placed above or to either side of the area that is giving pain, and the results are felt straight away. TENS can be used to manage both acute and chronic pain but may not work for everyone. For people with pacemakers, women in the first 3 months of pregnancy and people who operate heavy machinery, TENS is not an appropriate form of pain relief.

If it is appropriate for you, your GP can refer you to a hospital physiotherapy department or a community physiotherapist who will be able to loan you a TENS machine for several weeks. If TENS is effective in reducing your pain, you may wish to buy your own machine (high street chemists and Argos stock TENS equipment).

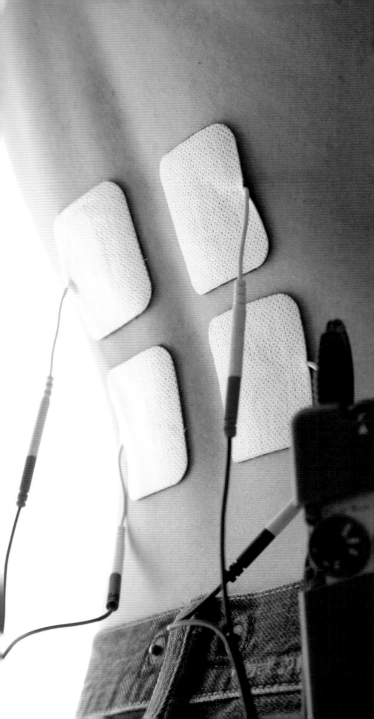

## Back schools

After 8 weeks, 70% of people who went to back school felt that their back pain had got better. After 6 months, 40% still felt better.

Back schools – classes taught by physiotherapists or doctors – teach people with chronic back pain how their backs work, what causes their pain and offer them advice about staying active. Educating people about how mechanical strain and bad posture can worsen their pain, and showing them the correct way to lift objects, to get in and out of bed or to stand properly, allows them to adapt their lives to reduce their pain and prevent future back problems. Whilst back schools may be effective in the short term, at the moment it is not clear whether their positive-effects results extend beyond 12 months. Your GP will be able to advise you of back schools in your local area.

## Acupuncture

'Acupuncture' comes from the Latin 'acus' (meaning 'needle') and 'pungere' (meaning 'prick').

Acupuncture is an ancient Chinese medical treatment that relieves pain and cures disease through the insertion of very fine needles into the body at specific points. There are around 500 acupuncture points all over the body. By mapping 'energy pathways' throughout the body, acupuncture affects the functioning of certain organs in the body. However, the area that is stimulated by the needle may not necessarily be close to the part of the body where you are experiencing pain. For example, even though you are suffering from headaches, needles may be inserted in your foot or hand.

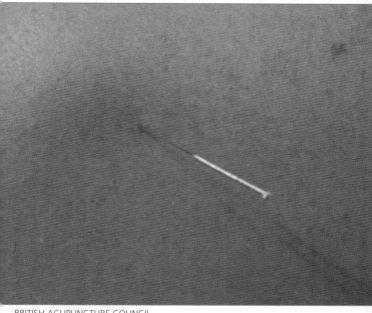

BRITISH ACUPUNCTURE COUNCIL.

At your first consultation, an acupuncturist
will ask you about your symptoms, your
medical history and your health in general.
They may also feel the quality, rhythm and
strength of the pulses on both of your wrists.
It is important that you choose an
acupuncturist who is suitably qualified. The
British Acupuncture Council
(*www.acupuncture.org.uk*) will be able to
advise you.

**BACK SURGERY**

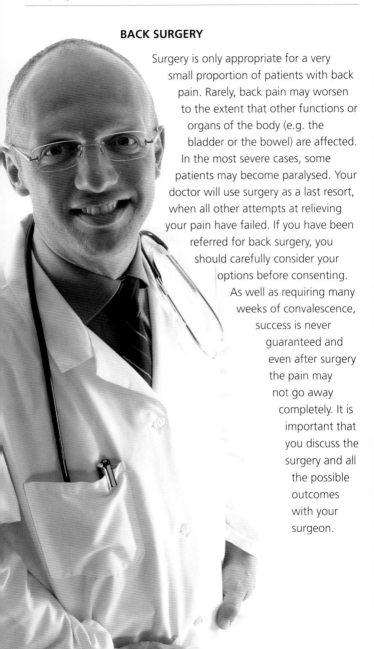

Surgery is only appropriate for a very small proportion of patients with back pain. Rarely, back pain may worsen to the extent that other functions or organs of the body (e.g. the bladder or the bowel) are affected. In the most severe cases, some patients may become paralysed. Your doctor will use surgery as a last resort, when all other attempts at relieving your pain have failed. If you have been referred for back surgery, you should carefully consider your options before consenting. As well as requiring many weeks of convalescence, success is never guaranteed and even after surgery the pain may not go away completely. It is important that you discuss the surgery and all the possible outcomes with your surgeon.

Useful questions to ask your back pain specialist include:

- what kind of operation are you proposing?
- what are the chances of good pain relief if I opt to have the surgery?
- what will happen if I decide not to have the surgery?
- what are my other options besides surgery?
- what are the possible risks associated with this kind of surgery?
- how long will I be in hospital for?
- will I have to undergo physiotherapy after the operation?
- how long will I have to stay off work?
- how long after the surgery will my life return to normal?

There are three general types of back surgery:

- discectomy – involves the removal of part of a vertebral disc to reduce pressure on a nerve root
- decompression – involves the removal of tissue that is compressing a nerve and disturbing major functions like the control of the bladder or bowels
- stabilisation/fusion – involves fixing together two or more adjacent vertebrae with bone taken from elsewhere in the body.

## SPECIAL TREATMENT GROUPS

### Back pain and pregnancy

Back pain during pregnancy is a relatively common problem. The growing foetus may cause postural problems and, towards the end of the pregnancy, the position of the baby can compress nerves and cause back pain this way. The hormones you produce whilst you are pregnant can also affect your back. Some pregnancy hormones cause the ligaments between the pelvic bones to soften and your joints to loosen in preparation for the birth. As the structures that support your pelvic organs become more flexible, you may feel considerable discomfort on either side of your lower back.

There are a number of steps that women can take to avoid back pain whilst they are pregnant:

- wear low-heeled shoes with good arch support
- sleep on your side with a pillow between your legs
- use a support belt to take some of the weight of your baby away from your back
- avoid slouching wherever possible

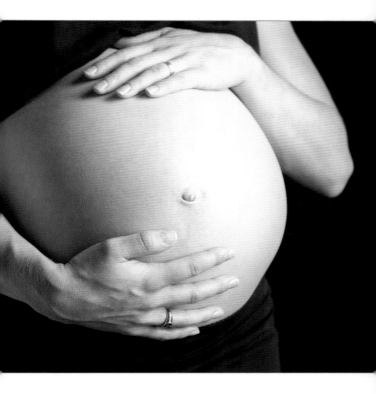

- avoid bending over with your legs straight (and placing excessive strain on your lower back)
- do pelvic tilts to strengthen the pelvis and reduce lower back pain
- take warm baths or use a warm jet of water from a shower head
- exercise regularly (but always consult your doctor before starting any exercise routine).

## Can I take painkillers whilst I am pregnant?

Being pregnant may affect which types of analgesic you can take safely without causing harm to your baby. Paracetamol is not known to be harmful in pregnant women and is usually preferred over other painkillers. In contrast, aspirin and ibuprofen are not recommended, especially in the later stages of pregnancy. Some clinical studies have even linked the use of these drugs with an increased chance of miscarriage. Your doctor will not usually prescribe opioids as pain relief whilst you are pregnant. If you already take prescribed opioids and you are planning to get pregnant, you should seek medical advice before trying to conceive. Your doctor will weigh up the risks to you and to your baby and may suggest alternative pain medications. This is because babies of women taking opioids have about a 50% chance of showing symptoms of drug withdrawal after birth.

## Back pain and the elderly

Elderly people are more likely to experience vertebral fractures as a result of underlying, age-related bone diseases such as osteoporosis. For this reason, they may require more pain relief than people of a younger age. The painkillers aspirin and other NSAIDs (e.g. ibuprofen) should be used with caution in the elderly. This is because older people are more susceptible to the side-effects of these drugs, like increased gastrointestinal bleeding and abdominal pain.

Before resorting to these drugs, it is advisable to try other means of pain relief if possible. These may include losing weight, using a walking stick and keeping warm, and in terms of drugs, using paracetamol instead of aspirin, or using a low dose of ibuprofen. Another option is combining paracetamol with a weak opioid analgesic.

## THE LONG AND THE SHORT OF IT

### What should I expect?

Realistically speaking, if you have suffered from back pain in the past, the chances are that you will suffer from it again. Up to 80% of people who have had back pain will get it again within a year. The trick is to learn how to handle and stay in control of your back pain, either by anticipating and preventing it, or by learning to live with it. Remember, in the vast majority of cases, back pain lasts for less than 2 weeks.

### Will it go away on its own?

In all probability, your back pain will sort itself out. If it doesn't then there are a number of things you can try that may relieve your pain. Although a complete cure may be difficult to achieve, you should be able to live with your back pain without it restricting your lifestyle significantly. Most importantly, you should not allow pain to control the way in which you live your life.

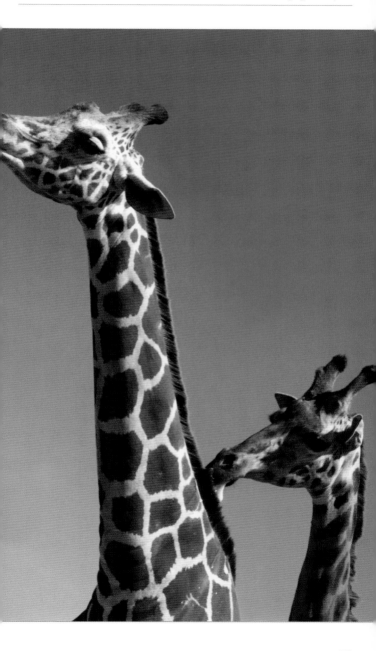

**BECOMING AN EXPERT PATIENT**

Back pain is a long-term condition that usually recurs throughout life. People with back pain may benefit from joining the Expert Patient Programme, run by the NHS. The scheme is aimed at encouraging people with long-term health conditions to take more control over their health by understanding and managing their conditions. By enrolling on the Expert Patient Programme you will ultimately be able to use your skills and knowledge to lead a fuller life. Courses take 6 weeks to complete and are run throughout the country. Visit *www.expertpatients.nhs.uk* for more information.

**FIVE STEPS TO GETTING THE MOST OUT OF YOUR HEALTH SERVICE**

**1** Maintain a good relationship with your GP and the other members of your team.

**2** Keep your team informed of any changes you notice in your symptoms.

**3** Keep your team informed of all the treatments you are taking.

**4** Agree with your team on your personal management targets.

**5** Know what to expect and when you need to ask for help.

## GETTING THE MOST OUT OF YOUR HEALTH SERVICE

If you have had one episode of back pain, the chances are that you will experience another at some point later in your life. Back pain can be a long-term condition and it needs to be treated on a case-by-case basis. Maintaining a good relationship with your GP, or any other member of your pain management team, is fundamental to managing your back pain effectively. These people will be able to explain to you why you are in pain, teach you how best to manage your pain or to avoid it in the first place, and help to relieve your pain by physical manipulation, drug treatment, or in the most severe cases, surgery.

It is important that you remain in regular contact with a member of your pain management team, keeping them informed of any improvement or deterioration in your pain control. Remember, if one management approach fails to work, there are many others that can be tried.

Visiting your doctor can sometimes be a confusing or daunting prospect. You may find that the consultation flies by and when your doctor asks if you have any questions, your mind goes blank. Writing down a list of questions before the consultation, may help you to get the most out of your appointment.

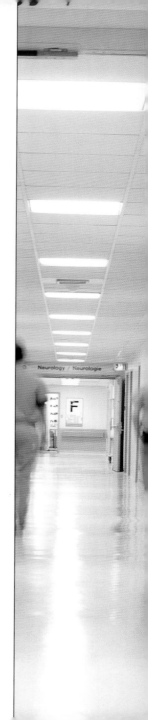

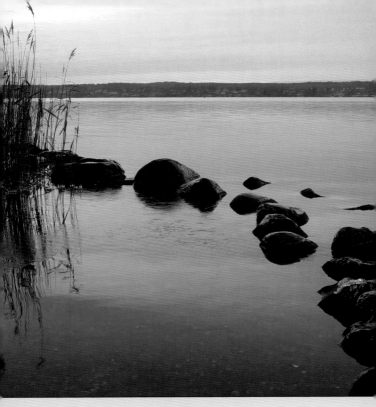

## QUESTIONS TO ASK YOUR DOCTOR

- Do you know what's causing my back pain?
- How severe is my back pain?
- It is likely to get worse?
- Do I need to have any tests?
- What type of treatment suits me best?
- What should I do if the treatment doesn't make me feel better?
- Can I carry on going to work?
- How long will it take for me to get better?
- What else can I do to make my back feel better?
- Are there any exercises that can make my back stronger?
- Are there any alternative or complementary therapies that might help?
- What can I do to avoid getting back pain again?
- Is it all right for me to drive?

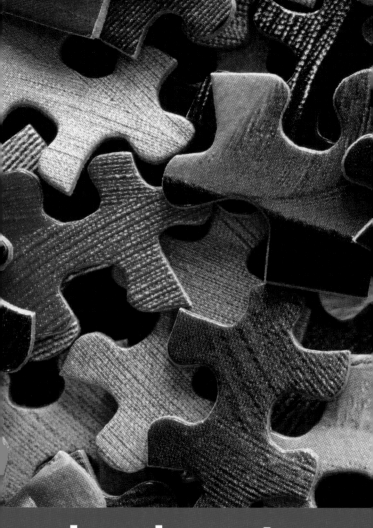

# simple extras

## FURTHER READING

- *BESTMEDICINE Osteoporosis* (2005)
  240pp, ISBN: 1-905064-81-0, £12.95
  Website: *www.bestmedicine.com*

## USEFUL CONTACTS AND ADDRESSES

- **Arthritis and Musculoskeletal Alliance**
  Bride House
  18–20 Bride Lane
  London
  EC4Y 8EE
  Website: *www.arma.uk.net*
  Tel: 020 7842 0910/11
  Email: *arma@rheumatology.org.uk*

- **BackCare**
  16 Elmtree Road
  Teddington
  Middlesex
  TW11 8ST
  Website: *www.backcare.org.uk*
  Tel: 020 8977 5474

- **Best Treatments UK**
  Website: *www.besttreatments.co.uk/btuk*

- **British Acupuncture Council**
  63 Jeddo Road
  London
  W12 9HQ
  Website: *www.acupuncture.org.uk*
  Tel: 020 8735 0400
  Email: *info@acupuncture.org.uk*

■ **British Brain and Spine Foundation**
7 Winchester House
Cranmer Road
Kennington Park
London
SW9 6EJ
Website: *www.bbsf.org.uk*
Helpline: 0800 808 1000
Tel: 020 7793 5900

■ **British Pain Society**
21 Portland Place
London
W1B 1PY
Website: *www.britishpainsociety.org*
Tel: 020 7631 8871

■ **Chartered Society of Physiotherapy**
14 Bedford Row
London
WC1R 4ED
Website: *www.csp.org.uk*
Tel: 020 7306 6666

■ **General Chiropractic Council**
44 Wicklow Street
London
WC1X 9HL
Website: *www.gcc-uk.org*
Tel: 020 7713 5155
Email: *enquiries@gcc-uk.org*

■ **General Osteopathic Council**
176 Tower Bridge Road
London
SE1 3LU
Website: *www.osteopathy.org.uk*
Tel: 020 7357 6655
Email: *info@osteopathy.org.uk*

■ **The Health and Safety Executive**
Rose Court
2 Southwark Bridge
London
SE1 9HS
Website: *www.hse.gov.uk* / *www.hse.gov.uk/betterbacks*
Tel: 020 7717 6000.
Information Line: 0845 345 0055

■ **NHS Direct**
Website: *www.nhsdirect.nhs.uk/*

■ **Pain Association Scotland**
Cramond House
Cramond Glebe Road
Edinburgh
EH4 6NS
Website: *www.painassociation.com/*
Tel: 0800 783 6059

- **Pain Relief Foundation**
  Clinical Sciences Centre
  University Hospital Aintree
  Lower Lane
  Liverpool
  L9 7AL
  Website: *www.painrelieffoundation.org.uk/*
  Tel: 0151 529 5820
  Email: *secretary@painrelieffoundation.org.uk*

- **The Patients Association**
  PO Box 935
  Harrow
  Middlesex
  HA1 3XJ
  Helpline: 0845 608 4455
  Tel: 020 8423 9111
  Website: *www.patients-association.com*

- **Spinal Injuries Association**
  Acorn House
  387–391 Midsummer Boulevard
  Milton Keynes
  MK9 3HP
  Website: *www.spinal.co.uk*
  Helpline: 0800 980 0501

- **For a list of specialised pain clinics in the UK**
  *www.tamethepain.co.uk*

## YOUR RIGHTS

As a patient, you have a number of important rights. These include the right to the best possible standard of care, the right to information, the right to dignity and respect, the right to confidentiality and underpinning all of these, the right to good health.

Occasionally, you may feel as though your rights have been compromised, or you may be unsure of where you stand when it comes to qualifying for certain treatments or services. In these instances, there are a number of organisations you can turn to for help and advice. Remember that lodging a complaint against your health service should not compromise the quality of care you receive, either now or in the future.

■ **Patients Association**
The Patients Association (*www.patients-association.com*) is a UK charity which represents patient rights, influences health policy and campaigns for better patient care.
**Contact details:**
PO Box 935
Harrow
Middlesex
HA1 3YJ
Helpline: 08456 084455
Email: *mailbox@patients-association.com*

■ **Citizens Advice Bureau**
The Citizens Advice Bureau (*www.nacab.org.uk*) provides free, independent and confidential advice to NHS patients at a number of outreach centres located throughout the country (*www.adviceguide.org.uk*).
**Contact details:**
Find your local Citizens Advice Bureau using the search tool at *www.citizensadvice.org.uk*

- **Patient Advice and Liaison Services (PALS)**
  Set up by the Department of Health (*www.dh.gov.uk*), PALS
  provide information, support and confidential advice to patients,
  families and their carers.
  **Contact details:**
  Phoning your local hospital, clinic, GP surgery or health centre
  and ask for details of the PALS, or call NHS Direct on 0845 46 47.

- **The Independent Complaints Advocacy Service (ICAS)**
  ICAS is an independent service that can help you bring about
  formal complaints against your NHS practitioner. ICAS provides
  support, help, advice and advocacy from experienced advisors
  and caseworkers.
  **Contact details:**
  ICAS Central Team
  Myddelton House
  115–123 Pentonville Road
  London N1 9LZ
  Email: *icascentralteam@citizensadvice.org.uk*
  Or contact your local ICAS office direct.

**Accessing your medical records**

You have a legal right to see all your health records under the Data
Protection Act of 1998. You can usually make an informal request to
your doctor and you should be given access within 40 days. Note
that you may have to pay a small fee for the privilege.

You can be denied access to your records if your doctor believes
that the information contained within them could cause serious
harm to you or another person. If you are applying for access on
behalf of someone else, then you will not be granted access to
information which the patient gave to his or her doctor on the
understanding that it would remain confidential.

**PERSONAL RECORD:**

**My Simple Guide**

This Simple Guide to Back Pain belongs to:

Name:

Address:

Tel No:

Email:

In case of emergency please contact:

Name:

Address:

Tel No:

Email:

**My Healthcare Team**

GP surgery address and telephone number

Name:

Address:

Tel No:

I am registered with Dr

My physiotherapist

My neurosurgeon

My pharmacist

Other members of my healthcare team

**QUESTIONS**

_____

_____

_____

_____

_____

_____

_____

_____

_____

_____

_____

_____

_____

_____

_____

_____

**ANSWERS**

_____

_____

_____

_____

_____

_____

_____

_____

_____

_____

_____

_____

_____

_____

_____

_____

_____

_____

**NOTES**

_____

_____

_____

_____

_____

_____

_____

_____

_____

_____

_____

_____

_____

_____

_____

**NOTES**

**NOTES**

_____

_____

_____

_____

_____

_____

_____

_____

_____

_____

_____

_____

_____

_____

**NOTES**

**NOTES**